A CHRISTIAN YOGA PRACTICE

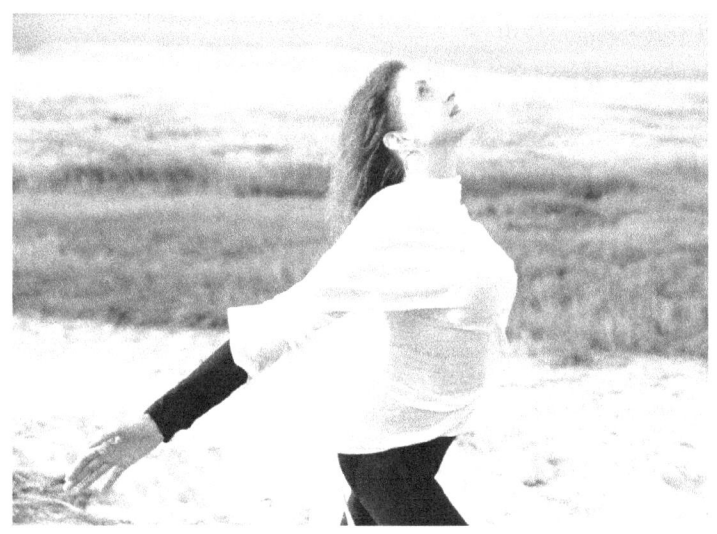

Befriending the SOUL of the Body

Marsha Therese Danzig

M.Ed Harvard

1

Table of contents

Welcome

Welcome to a Christian Yoga Practice!

This book is dedicated to LOVE, the love that I have found through a real, ongoing spiritual relationship with Jesus. I consider Jesus my greatest ally, friend, confidante, healer, sustainer and reminder of the beauty in each day. My own personal story is like so many who will be restored through this book: I have experienced so much heartbreak in this lifetime, and have been resurrected over and over to the grace of knowing God's loving presence. Miracles large and small happen so often I have lost count. It is through this Christ that we have an opportunity to see the fullness of life, our being , our light, our purpose, our security, our strength, our wisdom. It is in this human body here on earth that we articulate and manifest the message of HOPE that Jesus' life story offers. Eashoa Msheekhah is the Aramaic name for Jesus the Savior- The Anointed One, Life Giver ." I have come that you might have life and have it abundantly." Yoga has certainly brought the JOY of life to me in so many ways.

Love, Marsha

What miracles have happened today in your life?

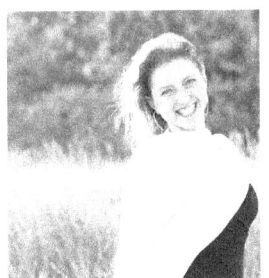

Yoga is the practice of living fully within body , mind , spirit and soul. Jesus' message is that through Faith, we are living fully in body, mind, spirit and soul. The old has passed away and all things have become new. Sometimes that is more of a belief than a physical reality. **The body is our great truth teacher.** Through Yoga, which looks at the body as a whole, we can access this truth on a very deep and integrated level, thereby bringing contentment in to our being, peace being directly manifested on all levels because we are all divinely connected and all children of God.

Yoga helps us align ourselves in the physical plane first through the practice of asana, or posture. This alignment of our bodies also addresses our emotions , spirit and soul. In other words, everything gets activated. Deep seated body messages of pain , stuckness, hurt, anger, close heartedness, and other traumas make way to new openings like compassion, grace, enthusiasm for life, freedom from pain, release from congested or blocked energy in the body. This practice completes the process by allowing the Holy Spirit, the Healer and the Great Physician to complete this good work in you on all levels. It is said " By His Stripes we have been healed". And so, the 'work' of yoga, the deep penetrating processes are a discovery of the fact that we have already been healed which is now in our conscious, awakened state. Thus there is nothing to achieve in yoga. There is only THIS moment of grace, this moment of complete fullness. This is why Christ said not to worry about tomorrow, for tomorrow will take care of itself. Many times what we think we are asking for is physical healing or answers to questions in our lives, guidance for our work, our relationships, our Divine purpose .By listening to the body through meditative, prayerful devotional yoga practice, we may be led in to an even more abundant understanding of the questions as well as healing in ways we never imagined.

God wants the best for us. His/her whole purpose is wrapped up in loving us to be the Ones we were meant to be on this earth: to live in the Bliss of our individual Divine plan. We deeply access bliss through the practice of yoga.

Yoga, or union, is a term for an ancient esoteric practice. The original practice was done by hermits secluded from the world to meditate on the Divine, and to get in touch with the divine /pure state of being, thereby "yoking" the divine with their own humanity. The Christian perspective is that we are a reflection of the Divine , that God lives in us, but we are not , nor do we claim to be, God, but rather God's representatives here on earth , to spread the message of Christ's loving redemption.

By becoming aware of the body's sensations, the flux of energy and waves of feeling that emerge from the practice of yoga, we become tuned in to the guidance of the Holy Spirit. Jesus said to first love ourselves, then we are equipped to love others. It is through this deep practice of Self- inquiry that we become ready instruments for Christ. One perspective is that we are spiritual beings on a human journey, that the whole of our life journey is simply a remembering of who we ARE in God, that every new 'discovery' is actually just another expression of awakened consciousness. In Christ we are full , complete, healed, saved, forgiven, in Sacred Unity with Christ. The good work we do on this earth comes from a place of wholeness, not fearful duty, and flows from us effortlessly because we are in the FLOW of the Holy Spirit.

Get in to the flow .

Becoming quiet .

Listening to the voice
within.

Be still, and know that I

*Yoga practice is a prayer which will support
us in all realms of our life.*

Strength for challenging situations.
Flexibility with decision making.
Openness with others and ourselves.
Peace in the midst of the storm.
Unity with all beings on the earth.
Harmony within ourselves.
Wisdom to know our inner guidance.
Trust when we can't see ahead .
Faith in life.
Space for our mistakes.
Gratitude for the gifts in our life.
Respect for the human body's journey.
Love , both received and given.

Journal Questions

Why do you want to practice yoga?

What do you believe you will gain?

How can yoga bring you closer to God?

Yoga Basics

Yoga is an ancient form of healing that goes back thousands of years. It originates in India. One of the first recorded documents came by way of *Patanjali*, who wrote the Sutras, (sayings, or threads) and meditations on the different aspects of yoga. Most importantly he introduced the eight limbed path of yoga, which is still taught in yoga schools today. It is through this eight limbed path of *Astanga* , or *Raja(Royal)Yoga* that we achieve Union with the Divine, or *Samadhi.* In a Christian Yoga practice, we observe the tenets this eight limbed path, knowing that we are ALWAYS in union with Christ at any stage of the path. We have all become kings and queens on the royal path when we believe that the kingdom of God is within our hearts, minds, bodies and spirits.

The eight limbed path, or Astanga includes:

Yama-*ethics*

Niyama - *purity and self- care*

Pranayama -*mastery/control of prana (life energy)*

Asana- *yoga postures*

Pratyahara -*withdrawal of senses*

Dharana -*concentrated focus*

Dhyana -*deep meditation*

Samadhi- *complete absorption in to the Absolute*

It is through the first four limbs that we begin to hone our spiritual skills by addressing the Physical body. With continued practice, this skill will becomes second. The body is the messenger, and although we wait with much anticipation for our physical bodies to be transformed into fully realized bodies with our death, we are here, on this earth

15

NOW. NOW is always. Take Christ's words seriously when He tells us that He came so that we might have life abundantly in the NOW, here, present.

The basis for yoga is the breath. Pranayama, the second limb of the Astanga yoga, is the practice of breathing, in all different ways, to bring about different experiences. The magic of Pranayama practice is that often, within seconds, we begin to experience levels of peace, calm, connection, and stress reduction. This is very exciting, because in this too we are given an experience of God, who is the breath behind our breath. Best of all, this is available for us ALL THE TIME. Pranayama provides a direct link to Our Creator and can reassure us of His presence when we are struggling, sick, worried, grieving, and alone.

From the practice of Pranayama we move in to *Asana*. Asana is the physical practice of Yoga. Asana can be translated as "sitting in the consciousness of God". When we are in our posture, positioned in our seat, we observe the state of our breath, our bodies, our emotions, our mental states, and our spirit. We observe areas of balance. Harmony, integration and we compassionately address those parts of ourselves that feel Out of balance, disharmonious, non-integrated. We lovingly embrace the whole of ourselves. We celebrate exactly who we are on the yoga mat and off the yoga mat. We acknowledge the Grace of God who sees our efforts.

There comes a point in a posture when effort ceases, when the mind/body/spirit feels aligned, harmonious. This is just another level of consciousness. There is nothing to achieve in yoga, as in Christianity. We are already in God, already loved and forgiven. There are only lesser and greater degrees of conscious awareness of this reality.

16

Whoever drinks this water I give him will never thirst. Indeed, the water I give him will become in him a spring of water welling up to eternal life." John 4: 14.

Asana gives way to **withdrawal of senses, or** *Pratyahara*. As we delve deeper and deeper in to the yoga posture, we withdraw from the exterior sensations and connect to the Well of Living Water that dwells within us. This also is Christ.

From Pratyahara, **we go to** *Dharana*, **or focused attention.** We can think of this as the direct intentional observance of the energetic experiences brought on by yoga practice. We become aware of the subtleties of the body, mind and spirit. We begin to feel and see that this body is not just physical matter, but is actually worlds of spinning energy, being held together by this greater web, which again is God breathing in to us and making us whole.

Dharana leads to *Dhyana*, **or meditation,** when the self can begin to transform the busy thoughts of the mind and merge with the Light of the divine. Meditation is the steady internal observance of the present moment, **BEING in God Rather than DOING for God.** When we begin to understand that each moment is an eternal moment we can live more fully in our lives, therefore being FULL of the love of Christ.

Finally we have *Samadhi*, **or Blissful union with the divine,** which brings us back to the word Yoga, or Yoke. A yoke is a restraint that allows animals to pull wagons in harmony. Without a yoke, the animals can become exhausted as they struggle to plow a field. Farmers often yoke an experienced animal with a less experienced animal so that the less experienced animal can learn to walk more in unison.

Jesus is there, yoked eternally to us, leading us on until we are on equal footing so can walk triumphantly through our battles, our suffering, and our life. To know too that we are on equal footing with Christ in this life is very reassuring. This occurs because *"the Word Became Flesh and made His dwelling among us." John 4:14.* Hallelujah!

There have been many yogis and Christian mystics who have experienced this divine union, this state of Bliss. I believe they were experiencing Christ, but did not know Him as Christ. This is also available to us. There is nothing we need to achieve or perform. We are God's children, so we can simply ask for what we desire from this Loving Father/ Mother.

" Come to me for
my yoke is easy
and my burden is
light"

Journal Questions

Meditation: Are you comfortable with meditation? Why or why not?

Bliss: Do you believe God wants us to experience bliss?

What IS Yoga?

There are many types of YOGA being practiced today. Some examples are:

- **Bhakti-** The Yoga of Devotion to God
- **Karma-** The Yoga of Selfless Service
- **Hatha-** The Yoga of Physical Practice
- **Jnana-** The Yoga of Scripture Study
- **Raja-** The Eight Limbed Path

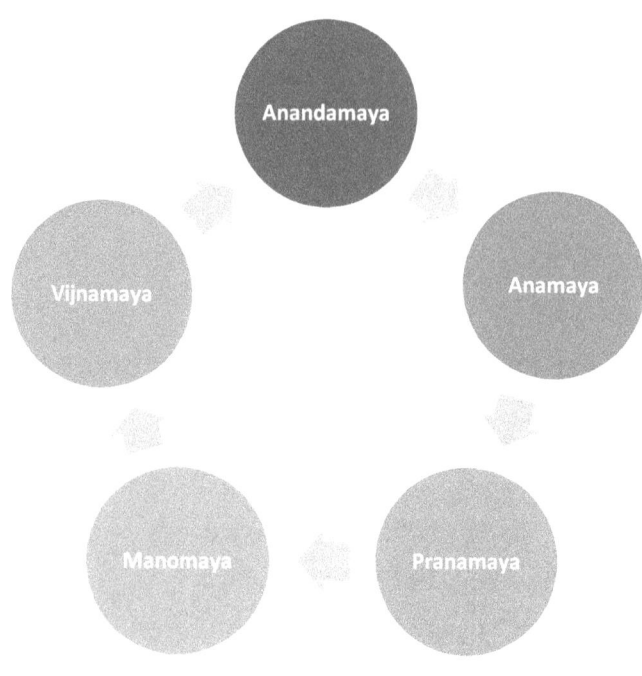

Within the esoteric principles of yoga there are considered to be 5 bodies, sheaths (koshas).

1) **Anamaya Kosha-** Food Sheath
2) **Pranamaya Kosha-** Breath Sheath
3) **Manomaya Kosha-** Mental Sheath
4) **Vijnanamaya Kosha-** Intellect Sheath
5) **Anandamaya Kosha-** Bliss Sheath

The sheaths can be looked at holographically, thus all the sheaths are interwoven .Harmony in one sheath means harmony in all sheaths. The same is true for disharmony. In the original Aramaic spoken by Christ, Jesus calls God Spirit- *"God is Spirit and his worshippers must worship Him in Spirit and Truth. "* John 4:24. 'God is Spirit- Allah Ha Ruach. Allah Ha- 'No-one and nothing is Excluded' in 'Ruach- Breath, or Spirit'.

When we take a leaf from a tree, the entire imprint and shape of the tree is holographically seen within the leaf. The leaf, then, is the tree and vice versa. So too with the sheaths. God can heal within any layer of our experience and it will affect the entire person Taken to the full, when an individual is healed within herself, she is likewise healing humanity and the planet. The ancient yogis understood that everything has a cause and effect. Loving the self, respecting the self, IS loving the world.

The concept of sound is the foundation of yoga. Behind all of Raja Yoga, behind the breath and the postures and the meditation is the SOUND. Yogis practiced chanting the sound of OM, which they believe to be the sound behind all sounds. Their study and observances led them to the conclusion that SOUND is the generator of all living things, that sound/vibration, is the web of life that holds everything together.

"In the beginning was the Word, the Word was with God and the Word Was God." John 1:1, 2. Jesus

Christ IS the sound behind all sounds, the vibration that made all things. We, in our bodies, are made of sound, vibrations coming together to form flesh. We know this through quantum physics. Matter can be broken down into the smallest and smallest form, and just as we can expand endlessly in to the universe, there is also no end to the tiniest of particles .Everything is sound. When we are in harmony, literally, in body, mind, spirit, soul, the vibration or frequency of our being is very high, and therefore more in alignment with that of the original SOUND, which is Christ incarnate. Therefore we work with the sheaths in yoga to bring about this divine alignment.

From the inner Kingdom of God come the sounds of our heart.

What we say from our source has energy. If we speak with love and care to ourselves, the body hears it. If we speak with criticism and judgment, again the body is now criticized and judged, and so a pattern of blocked energy is created. Sound is very powerful.

Within the body are several *nadis,* or rivers, some physical, such as the circulatory system and the spine (nervous system).There are other tributaries which are non-physical and have to do with the directional flow of energy, such as acupuncture points. Yoga works with all of these nadis to create vibrant energy and health, as well as equanimity in all circumstances: that is, a deep sense of peace.

Journal Questions

What does a sheath mean to you?

What does sound mean to you?

Living Ethics
Of Yoga

Just as sound is the foundation of yoga, the Yamas and Niyamas, are the guides.

The Yamas are the principles that sustain our body, mind and spirit. The Niyamas are the actions that we take based on the principles of the yamas. Rather than Ten Commandments, these principles are ten inner suggestions to live a full life without the burden of guilt and constant self reprimand.

Ahimsa:
- Conscious awareness of our actions
- Non harm to self and others, including the natural world

Satya
- Honest, clear communication with love
- Truthful demeanor

Asteya
- What's mine is mine. What's yours is yours.
- Honoring time

Brahmacharya:
- Responsible sexuality
- A season of celibacy to focus on the spirit

Aparigraha
- Non attachment to outcome, people, places , ideas and things

- **Shaucha**
    - ○ Purity & Cleanliness
- **Santosha**
    - ○ Contentment & Gratitude
- **Tapas**
    - ○ Committed & Disciplined
- **Swadhyaya**
    - ○ Self Inquiry & Scripture Study
- **Ishwara-Pranidhana**
    - ○ Surrender to God & Letting Go

These Yamas and Niyamas can be practiced interchangeably with heartfelt intention and guidance through Scripture, prayer and the Holy Spirit. One Yama or Niyama may speak to you for a long period of time.

May your practice bring you ever closer to The One
Who loves you.
May those who practice with you come to know that love.

Journal Questions

What does non-violence mean to you?

Is the Bible a violent book? Why or why not?

Which yama pops out for you? Is there something you need to tell God?

Which niyama is easiest for you?

Which niyama is hardest for you?

Which niyama do you avoid?

Sacred Space

Spaciousness is a quality of God. Endless space is the vision of a curious child, learning with great enthusiasm about the world around her. Even the dark corners, the painful places, these too can be looked on with space, openness, acceptance. Space is LOVE.

When we see our bodies as spacious, this frees up the mind to be receptive to God's inner whispers. Sacred space starts from within, and then expands out to the world around you. This SPACE, this LOVE is always available. To know this requires practice and self-observation.

Because yoga means union, it is Sacred Union. God, Allah Ha (in Aramaic) is Sacred Unity. Elohim, one of the many Hebrew names for God, is roughly translated as the One and the Many. God is in all things and in all people.

Jesus says as much when he tells his disciples *"I was naked and you clothed me, I was hungry and you gave me food."* And Paul writes in 1 Corinthians 12: 12, 13 "The *body is one unit, though it is made up of many parts; and though all the parts are many, they form one body. So it is with Christ. For we were baptized by One Spirit- and we were all given the One Spirit to drink."*

Are you struggling with deep emotional and physical pain? Christ is in these dark, painful places as well. When we give our bodies space and time, held places begin to open up, shift, release, and let go. Each wave that flows in to your sacred space is also the ocean. Christ makes us whole

There are many practical ways that you can make your space a sacred one. It really does not matter where you are practicing. It is the intention and effort that matter. Most importantly it is YOU and what YOU bring to your practice.

Create Your Sacred Space:

- Dim the lights
- Play soft ,gentle music
- Keeping the space clear and uncluttered
- Be sure the floor is suitable to yoga, clean, and without any strong smells.
- Be certain the space is warm enough.
- Have a chair available if you need to lean on something.
- Greet yourself with warmth and love.
- Light a candle
- Create a ritual which will turn into a habit- your YOGA habit!
- Wear loose , comfortable clothing
- Buy a yoga mat, yoga blocks, blanket , bolster and yoga strap

In any yoga experience, strong emotions such as tears or laughter may occur during your practice.

Be aware of your needs. Have compassion with yourself. Slow down. Be in the sensation, as if your practice were timeless. Let your practice be a true refuge from the busy world. Laugh. Respect yourself. Be confident.

You are a child of God!

Journal Questions

What do you need right now?

How do you feel about respecting that need?

Find your Center

Centering sets the tone for your practice. Centering is a time to go inside, find your core, that place within that timeless, beyond the cares of the world, spacious, peaceful. Jesus often went off by himself to pray and be with God. *Sometimes we just need to be alone with our SELVES.* We can do this with centering.

Here are the steps to centering yourself.

- *Sit down* on your mat in a comfortable position, with legs crossed, spine erect ,eyes ½ open or closed.

- *Gaze inward* or at a particular point on the ground.

- *Hands come together in a prayer*, in front of the heart , thumbs gently pressing the sternum.

- *Check in* with yourself . How ARE you?

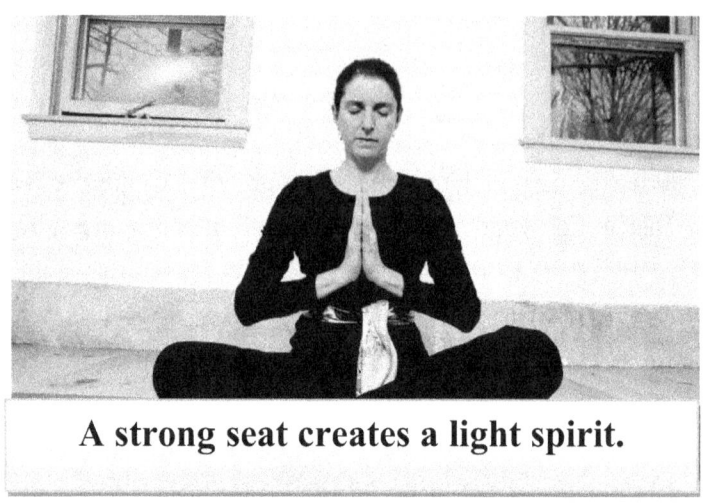

A strong seat creates a light spirit.

What are the benefits of centering?

Centering:

- Relaxes and calms the nervous system

- Clears the busyness of what came before ,making way for PRESENCE and BEING.

- Opens you to guidance from within, the gentle nudging of the Spirit.

- Gives you time to check in with yourself

  Take as much time as you need!

Centering techniques

Align	Pulling the flesh from your bottom diagonally out and sit cross legged
Body moves	Jiggle the body then relax with an "Aahhh."
Body scan	Notice how your body is feeling, head to toe.
Inner Space	Expand the SPACE of the heart to the edges of your body
Find the light	With each breath in, let the light in your heart get brighter. With each breath out, let that light fill you and grow larger
Tension/Release	Tighten parts of the body as you inhale, release with "AAHHH" as you exhale.
"I am " breath	Breathe in. Say to yourself "I". Breathe out say to yourself 'Am".
"This is me".	Take your right hand and tap gently on the heart center (thymus) silently chanting 'This is me" for several minutes.
Chant	A song or affirmation.
Meditate	Choose a word or phrase
Pray	See Chapter on Songs & Prayers

Journal Questions

How often do you feel centered in your life?

What do you gain from centering?

Which centering technique speaks to you? Why?

OM

Many Christians aren't sure how they feel about the sound of OM. It may feel sacrilegious or 'weird'. If this is you , simply avoid chanting Om.

I am a Christian who does chant Om. Let's look at the word, the sound and the meaning.

If you listen to the sound of Om , you hear echoes of Amen, Home, Mom. I believe that throughout the world, humanity is crying out to God, to know Him and to have answers to this life. We speak many languages in this world , and there are consequently many names for God. God, however in His infinite goodness and LOVE , speaks to us wherever we are .This means that Buddhists, Muslims, Sikhs and all faiths have deep and profound experiences of God. Anyone who is seeking God will find God.

"We know that the whole creation has been groaning as in the pains of childbirth right up to the present time." Romans 8:22. All roads ultimately lead to a crossroad. One is to continue on your present path if it is not with Christ, the other is to walk with Christ.

Om is a sound that is deeply embedded in our whole being. There is a sense of letting go in to the vastness of the ocean of God.

What does OM do?

- It relaxes the nervous system.

- It stimulates the Pineal gland, a Master Regulator gland.

- It awakens our spirit.

- It is calming and soothing.

Our whole body is formed by sound. When we use sound to center ourselves, our bodies come alive, with a deep memory of our infinite connection to the Divine.

What IS Om?

Om is a name for the Lord . Three letters make the symbol of Om. The A means "around". The U means "to put into". The M means "mmm". Combining these three letter and three sounds makes the sound of AUM, or Om.

The three letters that create the shape of Om represent the three aspects of God- Creator, Sustainer , Redeemer.

In the Hindu tradition, it is believed that the Lord created the world after chanting Om into the void, which is similar to the notion of "In the beginning was the Word." .

All prayers begin with Om. All great actions in the world begin with the chant of Om. Om sets the stage for viewing the world from holy eyes.

"A"(pronounced AAAHH.') is the *letting go*. An acknowledgement of ALLAH-HA. (God) .Primal energy. Possibility. Beginning. "U"(pronounced OOOOO) , a moving towards, from *unknown to known*, from the womb in to reality . "M"(pronounced MMMMMM), that which *purifies* creation, to life. Water of Life. The current of flow. Purification. God, being beyond vibration, has chosen to communicate to us through vibration.

Interestingly, it is said that these three sounds are **foundational sounds** in ALL languages. According to the Book of Genesis, at one time only one language was spoken.

Three is a number of great significance in the Bible. It stands for completion. Christ is part of the Trinity, the three persons of God in one. We can think of these three sounds as:

'A' Father/Mother/Creator

'U' Sustainer, Savior, Christ

'M' Holy Spirit, Mother/Father, Healer

Aaaaaa M En

Journal Question

How do YOU feel about OM?

Mudras

Mudras are hand gestures that can have symbolic, emotional, and real physical value. Our most familiar mudras are praying hands and the "Okay" gesture. When Jesus prayed for someone's healing , He more often than not used His hands to activate the prayer. There was a powerful exchange of energy at the onset of His prayers. In this chapter you will learn 7 simple mudras , along with their meaning , and an affirmation/prayer to accompany each one. Practice any time!

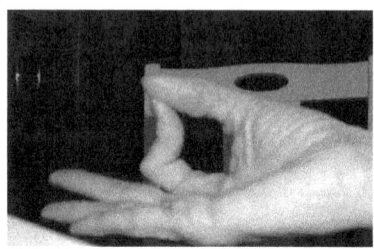

We begin with the symbol for "okay" which is also the symbol of Yoga, bringing together the individual self with the Highest Self, which is God, or uniting the known with the unknown, making them one. Everything is OKAY when you are yoked with God!

How to practice:

- *Bring the outer(index) and inner (thumb) together.*
- *Stretch remaining fingers out.*

When your fingers are pointing up, you are seeking Heaven. This is Gyan Mudra. When your fingers are down, you are seeking earth, This is Chin Mudra.

The Spirit of God dwells within me

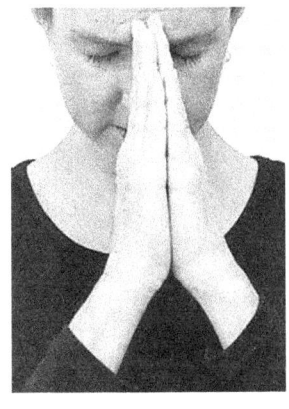

Prayer Mudra is used in all cultures of the world. Why would that be? The bringing together of the left hand with the right can be seen as the bringing together the male and female, the moon and sun, the hidden with the unhidden, the dark with the light. All comes together in front of and within the heart. Praying hands are reverent hands, reverence for the sacred place of the heart.

How to practice:

- *Press the right fingertips to the left fingertips.*
- *Press the heels of the hand together*
- *Gently press the palms together.*
- *Point the thumbs towards the heart or middle of the brow.*

All of my prayers have already been answered in Christ.

Peace Mudra is a peace offering. The palm is slightly rounded and soft, as if to say "I see you. I have my own boundaries as well, but I have room to welcome you in." I think of Jesus laying hands on people. A flat palm says "stay away", but a rounded palm creates both a sense of authority and grace.

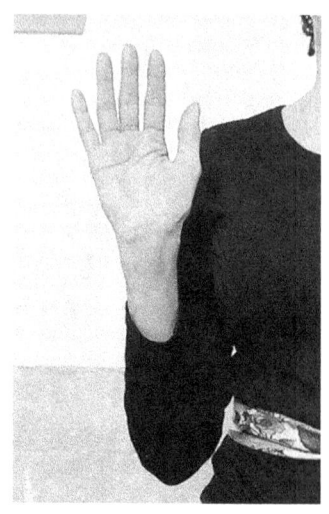

How to practice:

- *Bend right elbow at the ribs.*
- *Open palm with slight curve*
- *Fingers are relaxed and lifted*

I have been given a spirit of Strength.

Lotus Flower

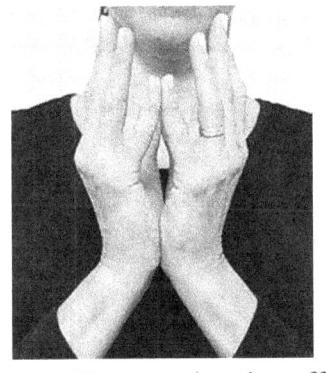

Lotus flower. This mudra forms an all embracing cradle around an open space, the budding womb of a flower. This is a mudra about becoming new "Behold all things have become new." In Christ we are a new creation, the old has passed away. When we practice the ***Niyama of Tapas,*** or burning off the old through intense effort, the hidden places (deep in the womb of our soul) can find their way to the surface and be offered up forever to God.

How to practice:

- *Press the wrists together with fingers pointing skyward.*
- *Touch the pinkies together & the thumbs together*
- *Form an open space in the center, as if holding a bud.*

I open to the possibilities of God.

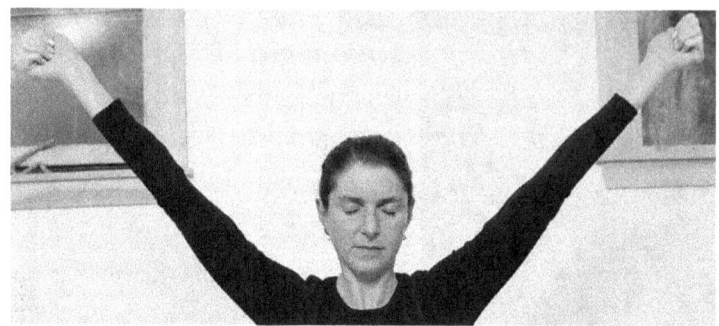

To life!   In this mudra we lift up the arms in a "V" and lift the thumbs up to heaven. This mudra is known as the "ego booster", as if to say, "thy will not mine, Lord, be done". It is a mudra of agreement with God, agreement with the bigger picture and a willingness to trust that God really does know what he is doing.

How to practice:

- *Lift arms up in a wide V*
- *Roll thumbs back and up*

I allow God to do His good work in me.

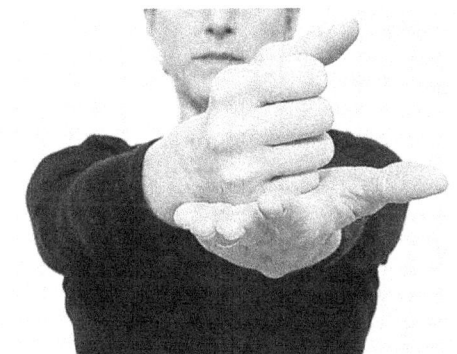

This mudra affirms our inner power. Many of us have been taught that we are unworthy and unlovable, even within the Christian church. When we believe those lies, we lose our power. The whole reason for Christ is not only to restore us but also to remind us of our goodness.

How to practice:

- *Outstretch the left arm with the palm up and flat*
- *Curl the right hand in to a gentle but firm fist*
- *Rest the right fist inside the left palm*
-

I have a right to be here because

I am God's child.

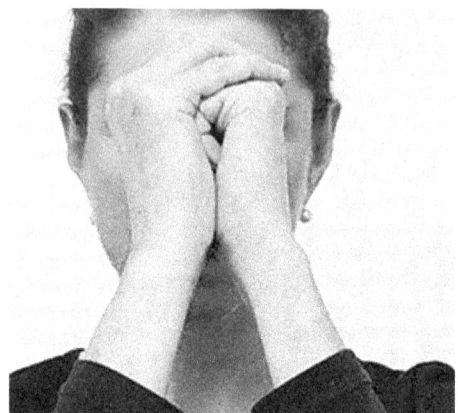

This mudra taps into our "third eye" or inner eye. There is a direct link between the midpoint of the brow point and the pineal gland in the brain, which is often referred to in yoga as the nectar of life. This nectar creates feelings of bliss and awareness.

How to practice:

- *Wrap the right hand over the left*
- *Press the thumbs together.*
- *Gently press the thumbs in to the brow point*

Jesus is my source.

Journal Questions

Where do you feel your purposes are aligned with God?

Where do you feel your purposes are out of alignment with God?

What affirmation speaks to you?

Which mudra is calling your name? Why?

How do you feel when you practice that mudra?

Pranayama

Pranayama or control of the life force(the breath) is THE basic building block of yoga practice. First we breathe, then we move. Without a focus on the breath, yoga becomes a form of stretching ,or acrobatics. It is only through the breath that we come to see yoga as a sacred experience, a remembering of the sanctity of this gift we call life. God is the breath behind our breath. Therefore when we breathe in and out we experience the unity that is within all things. All living things breathe. ALL.

The word for breathing in is inspiration.

We breathe in SPIRIT.

" Spirit of the living God, fall afresh on me."

Pranayama does not have to be complicated. As Jesus said, *"My yoke is easy, my burden is light."* Breath comes because we are a part of God. So breathe deep!

"Your workmanship is marvelous- and how well I know it, You were there while I was being formed in utter seclusion! You saw me before I was born and scheduled each day of my life before I began to breathe." Psalm 139: 15, 16.

In this chapter you will learn four basic breath techniques.

Dirgha : 3 part breath

We use all three parts of the torso to bring about deep, soothing, transformative breath. The breath is slow, deliberate, conscious, aware. Dirgha breath teaches you to breathe deep in to your diaphragm. It cleanses the lungs of stale air, and uses all three parts of the lungs.

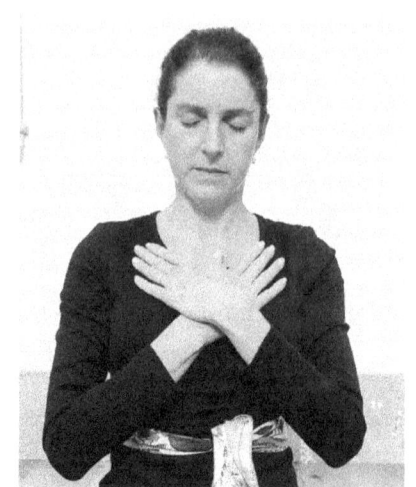

How to practice:

- *Inhale, the breath rising from the belly through the ribs and in to the chest.*

- *Exhale, the breath descending from the chest through the ribs to the belly.*

- *Lie down on your back with your knees bent, feet flat on the floor.*
- *Place your hands on your belly.*
- *Begin to breathe deeply, with mouth closed, lips soft, allowing breath to flow through the nostrils.*
- *Feel your belly rise and fall.*
- *Take your hands to your ribs.*
- *Breathe in and out through both nostrils.*
- *Take your hands to your upper chest, fingers resting lightly on the collar bone.*
- *Feel the chest expand and contract with each breath.*
- *Go back to your belly.*
- *As you inhale, slide your hands from the belly to the ribs to the chest.*
- *As you exhale, slide the hands down the chest through the ribs to the belly.*
- *As you inhale, silently say to yourself, Father, Son, Holy Spirit.*
- *As you exhale, surrender to God.*

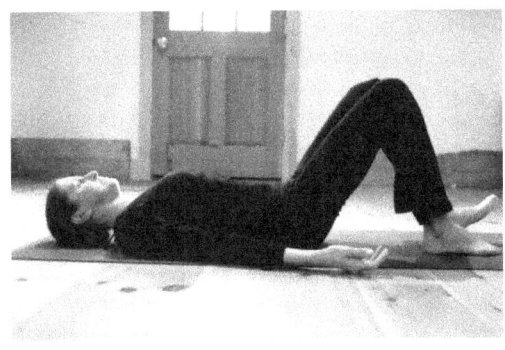

Ujjayi Pranayama.

Ujjayi Pranayama means breath of victory, because the sound of the breath can "overcome" the mind. This breath warms the body , focuses the mind and helps to deepen your postures.

"You are God, we shall do valiantly. It is He who will tread down our enemies."

How to practice:

- *Whisper the word "aaahhh" as you inhale and exhale, with your mouth closed*

- *Breathe through the back of the throat.*

- *Notice how warm the breath feels as if it were flooding your very bones with warm soothing oxygen.*

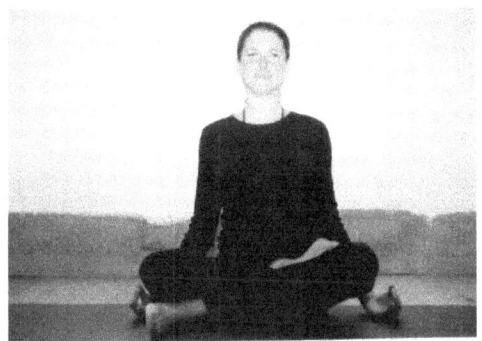

- *Sit up tall, legs in a comfortable position.*
- *Bring ALL your attention to your breath.*
- *Begin to practice Ujjayi breath with your eyes closed.*
- *Feel the texture of the breath as it enters your nostrils, moves down past your vocal cords and throat, on in to your body*
- *Notice where you feel the breath traveling.*
- *As you continue with each inhale and exhale, add a 1-2 second pause.*
- *This is the moment of possibility, the moment of creation, the moment that counts.*
- *Notice the quality of PRESENCE that can occur from just a few short breaths.*
- *This is Jesus, making Himself known to you .*
- *This peace and calm is ALWAYS available for you, for all of us.*

Nadi Shodhana

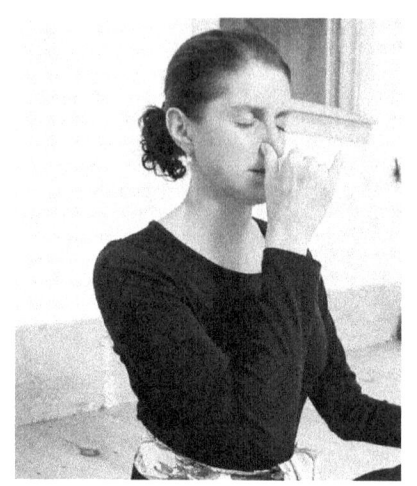

Nadi Shodhana means alternate nostril breathing. Nadi means channel and Shodhana means cleansing. This breath restores balance to the body, stimulating alternate sides of the brain. It is very calming, soft, and extremely gentle.

How to practice:

- *Take your right hand in to a mudra: thumb up, index finger and middle finger down, rind and pinky finger up.*

- *Take a deep breath in through both nostrils.*

- *Bring the right thumb to the right nostril.*

- *Exhale GENTLY through the left.*

- *Inhale through the left, close of this nostril with your pinky and ring finger as you open the right nostril to exhale.*

- *Exchange back and forth for a few rounds, ending with an exhale on the left side.*

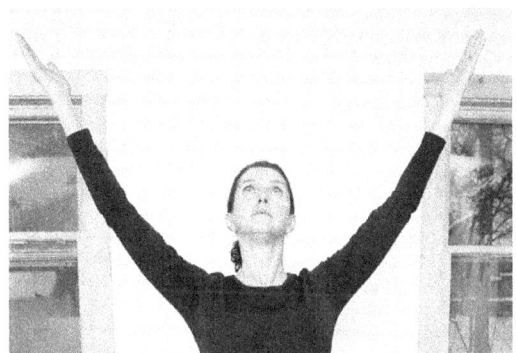

Son/Sun breath

Son/Sun breath is a circular movement of the arms from the sides of the body up overhead. This breath begins to prepare you for warm-ups and is an excellent to way stretch the side body.

How to practice:

- *Place the hands next to your side.*

- *Breathe in to your heart, recognizing the innate goodness within you and the blessing of being God's child.*

- *As you inhale, raise your arms up overhead until you are at your maximum level of inhale.*

- *Feel your arms being sustained by your breath, rather than your will.*

- *Before you release, be conscious of anything that has kept you from being fully in God.*

- *Let it go as you release your hands back to your side. Repeat as often as you like.*

Journal Questions

How is your breath like the Spirit of God?

How have you experienced victory in your life?

Pratapana

It is vitally important to warm up (pratapana) your body in preparation for asana (yoga poses). Choose one or two warm ups from each section. Practice warm-ups that work for you.

Foot and ankle warm ups:

- *Rotate ankles*
- *Hold ankle with hand and jiggle foot loosely*
- *Spread toes and place fingers between toes*
- *In standing position, curl toes under and up*
- *Massage feet*
- *Stomp feet*
- *Jump up and down*

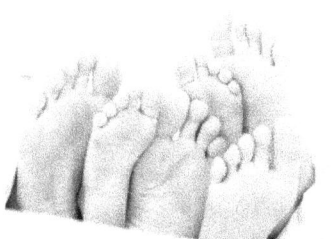

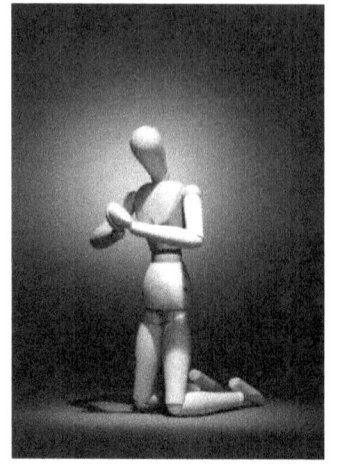

Knee Warm-ups

- *On back, hug knees in to chest*
- *On back, rest hands lightly on knees and take knees clockwise, then counter clockwise*
- *On back, draw knees apart and circle knees in opposite directions*
- *Sitting- draw feet together as knees spread apart(butterfly)*
- *Squat and twist, letting one knee touch the floor then the other*
- *Squat and lunge to one side then the other*

Legs/Hamstrings

- *On back, Take a strap and wrap around one leg, other leg extended. Draw circles with leg in strap. Switch legs.*

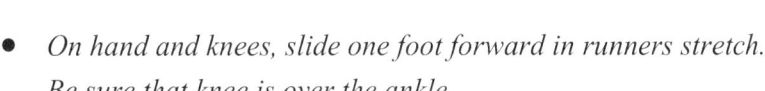

- *On hand and knees, slide one foot forward in runners stretch. Be sure that knee is over the ankle.*

- *Sitting, legs outstretched. Breathe in lift arms up. Breathe out bend over legs.*

- *Sit with feet pressed to wall and legs outstretched. Press in to wall as you lengthen the spine.*

- *Stand. Breathe in lift arms overhead. Breathe out bend forward gently.*

- *Downward Dog warm up. Come in to Downward dog. Bend right knee and press left heel down. Reverse.*

- *On back, draw one knee in to chest, while other leg is extended on floor Reverse.*

Hips

- *Sit cross legged. Place hands gently on knees. Take torso in a circle. Breathe in as you go back and breathe out as you go forward.*

- *Sit zig zag, right foot resting on left knee. Take left hand to left hip. Rock left hip back and forth. Reverse.*

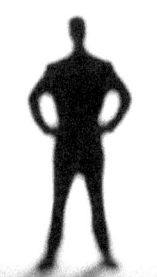

- *Sit zig zag. Place hands on either side of front knee. Inhale arch up and exhale round nose to knee. This is called dolphin.*

- *Stay in zig zag. Place hands behind bottom. Rock knees and hips from side to side.*

- *On back, knees bent. Cross right leg over left. Scoot hips to the right. Let knees fall to the left. Reverse.*

- *On Back, knees bent, feet on floor. Inhale lift bottom off floor. Exhale. Bring it back down.*

- *Stay on back and circle hips.*

- *On hands and knees and circle hips. Reverse circle.*

- *Stand feet hip width apart, hands on hips. Make hip circles.*

- *Sit cross legged. Grab hold of right leg and cradle in both arms Rock leg side to side. Reverse legs.*

Abdominals

- *On back, knees bent and feet at edge of mat. Reach hands between thighs as you exhale and lift torso with "Ha"*

- *On back. Knees bent. Feet on floor. Hands behind head. Inhale. Exhale lift head and chin off floor. Press abdominals in to floor.*

- *On hands and knees, Inhale draw right knee in to chest. Exhale kick it out behind you. Repeat on other side.*

- *Hands behind head, on back, Bicycle left and right. Twist elbow to meet opposite knee.*

- *On back, hands under sacrum, lift legs up and down.*

- *Standing. Knees slightly bent. Inhale. Extend right arm. Exhale, "Ha' as you pull it back to you, Reverse.*

- *Stand with knees slightly bent. Round over and rest hands on thighs. Breathe in, breathe out. Hold. Now pump the belly until the need for air is strong.*

Spine

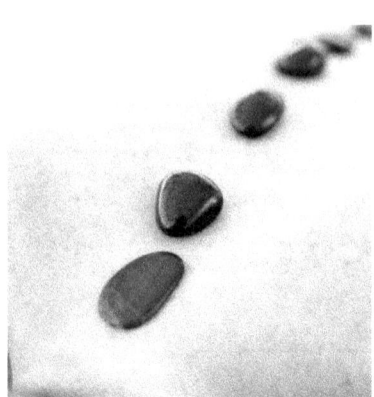

- *On back, knees bent, feet off floor. Sway knees to right as head turns to left. Reverse.*
- *Sitting cross legged, hands under shins. Inhale arch up, exhale round back*
- *Sitting cross legged. Inhale lengthen the spine exhale twist to the right – start from the belly. Rest right hand behind you on the floor.*
- *Lay on back, arms stretched overhead. Hook thumbs, Breathe in, hold, exhale completely.*
- *On hands and knees, arch like a cat(exhale) and extend like a cow(inhale)*
- *Spinal rocking- Hold knees. Rock back and forth.*
- *Stand tall. Begin to roll forward like a rag doll. Now roll back up.*

Shoulders

- *Sit cross legged. Draw right shoulder up to ear as you inhale. Circle back and down on exhale. Repeat on other side.*

- *Cross elbows and let hands rest on opposite shoulders. Inhale lift elbows up. Exhale. Relax Elbows down.*

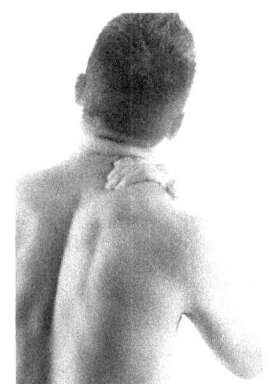

- *Eagle arms- cross left elbow over right. Bend elbows together .Cross left hand behind right. Reverse.*

- *Cow arms. Inhale as you draw left arm straight up. Right arm comes behind. Bend left elbow. Reach left hand for right hand. Repeat on other side.*

- *Standing. Take arms overhead in a V. vigorously criss-cross them, like flapping wings.*

- *Sitting or standing. Interlock hands behind sacrum. Squeeze hands down and back.*

- *Breath of Joy. In hale lift arms up overhead, inhale bring them to side, and then inhale again overhead. Now Exhale and fall forward limply with loose arms. "HHAAAA".*

- *Standing with strap. Make a wide V with strap. Reach to left and then to right.*

- *Interlock hands overhead. Reach to right then to left.*

Arms, Wrists, Hands

- *Reach both arms out, Circle wrists in both directions*
- *Standing. Swing arms from side to side*
- *Standing, Slide hands up to arm pits and down*
- *Sitting. Rub arms up and down, and then shake.*
- *Open left hand , palm up. Take right hand palm away and go between each finger. Draw the left fingers down with right hand. Reverse.*
- *Jiggle hands and fingers*

Fear not, for I am with you: be not dismayed, for I am God: I will strengthen you: I will help you: I will uphold you with my victorious right hand.
Isaiah 41:10

Head and Neck

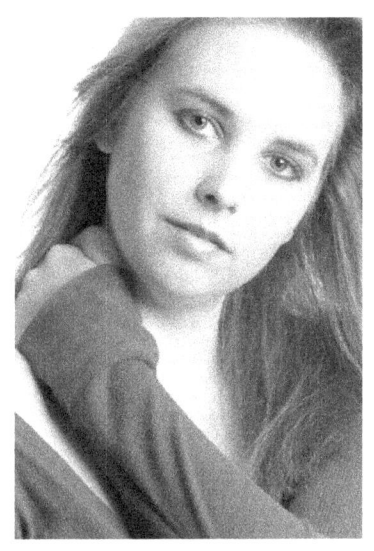

- *Inhale draw right ear to left shoulder. Exhale chin to chest. Inhale left ear to left shoulder.*

- *Turn head to right. Turn head to left.*

- *Cup back of head in hands. Arch back slightly with open mouth*

- *Interlock hands under chin. Draw elbows up and down as you inhale and exhale.*

- *Reach right arm out to right. Let right ear come to right shoulder. Bend right elbow and wrap around left ear. Repeat on other side.*

- *Shake head 'Yes' and 'No'*

Face

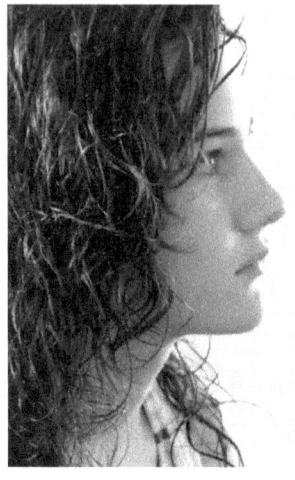

- *Tighten muscles on face as you inhale. Exhale relax face.*
- *Massage entire face including scalp.*
- *Tap point between eyebrows*
- *Rub hands together vigorously then cup over eyes for a few breaths*
- *Eye Clock. Move only your eyes as you "tell time"*
- *Dristi – gaze at a point in the distance – about 8-10 feet. Breathe slowly.*

With every warm-up we give consciousness to each part of the body. It is an honor to have this body. Warm up your body with appreciation for the One who made it.

Journal Questions

On what do you focus?

Do you take time to prepare or do you jump right in?

Is one way better than the other?

Why or why not?

Asana

Asana is the physical practice of yoga postures, which encourage strength, flexibility, poise, alignment, ease of breath, and healthy circulation. Translated as *"sitting in the consciousness of the Divine"*, Asana is the practice of removing obstacles in the body and mind that keep us separate from God. Once the pathways are clearer, the body more relaxed, the mind is then more receptive to hear God, be still, and know Him.

Asana is a practice of emancipation from our small self to be more of our true Self, who is the living reflection of God.

God created humans in His/her own image, in the image of God He/She created him; male and female He/She created them. Genesis 1:27

In asana, the soul shines through first, and from that radiant soul the pose emerges. This is why asana brings us so much into the present moment. With focus on our breath in each moment of the pose, we lose our distractions. We experience the fullness of the moment, which is full of God's potential in you.

Asana is a way to harness the energy already in our beings, to use it well, and efficiently. The spine creates the action. From that action, the body opens to the breath.

Tadasana

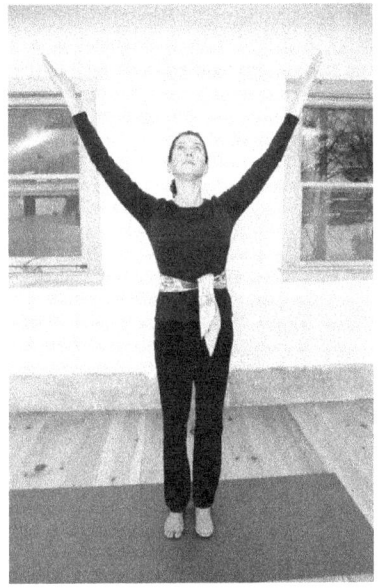

Mountain Pose

The Rock of My Refuge

Psalm 36:5-6

Your steadfast love reaches to the heavens
Your faithfulness to the skies
Your righteousness is like majestic mountains
And your wisdom like the depths of the sea

How to practice

- Stand with feet hip width apart
- Reach feet down into earth into all four corners as you lift crown up to the sky on exhale.
- Lift knee caps up
- Draw belly in
- Lift arms overhead on inhale, interlocking hands, index fingers pointing to the sky.

Variations

- Arms stay in T position
- Arms to side
- Palms in Namaste at heart center
- Toes together
- Stand against a wall for extra support
- Place yoga block between thighs to increase pelvic opening and stabilize core
- Interlock palms , turn up overhead
- Standing Backwards Prayer Pose. Place hands, palms together between the shoulder blades to expand the heart.

Benefits

- Great alignment positively affects EVERY system of the body. When the spine is erect, the head feels supported, the hips feel free yet grounded via the feet, every organ has space, nerves get relief, breath is easier, poise and grace follow you wherever you go, you stand in royalty
- Joints and bones of ankles, knees, shoulders, neck
- Develops stamina , strength and confidence
- Foundation pose for all standing Poses
- Creates peace lightness, awareness of body and breath,
- Balance

Contraindications

- Knee problems
- Shoulders or arm problems
- High blood pressure
- *Proceed with caution*- pregnancy, anxiety, serious heart problems, neck injuries, fibromyalgia(shorter holds)
- Recent knee surgery- keep knees soft

Vrikshasana

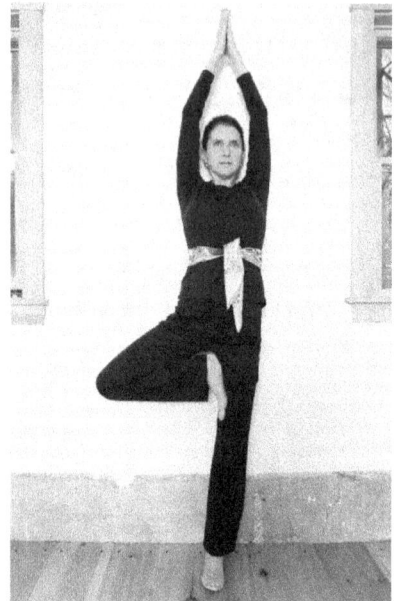

Tree Pose

The Vine

John 15:1-2

I am the true vine and

My Father is the gardener.

How to practice

- Stand in mountain
- Bend right knee, placing right foot to inside of inner left thigh or calf
- As you root down through the left leg, lift arms up overhead
- Lower right foot down
- Repeat on other side

Variations

- Keep arms to side, in a T, parallel to shoulders or in prayer position with the palms
- lean against a wall
- Stand side to side with a partner, opposite knees facing apart, tree trunks next to each other. Wrap arm around back of partner
- Keep foot on ground, just do turn out of knee and curl toes under near opposite foot
- Hold strap around bent leg

- Balance and coordination

- Spinal alignment

- Hip opener

- Strong ankles and legs

- Focus

- Peace

- Oblique muscles get stronger-can keep you from herniating

- greater lung capacity

- Observation of any imbalances in life brought to surface-emotional, physical, mental

- Circulation supported to become even better

- Leg muscles toned and strengthened

Contraindications/Cautions

- Knee surgery, inflammation, or recent injury

- Pregnancy or menses- practice with care

- High blood pressure

- Nerves and anxiety(practice shorter holds so as not to overstimulate system)

Five Pointed Star

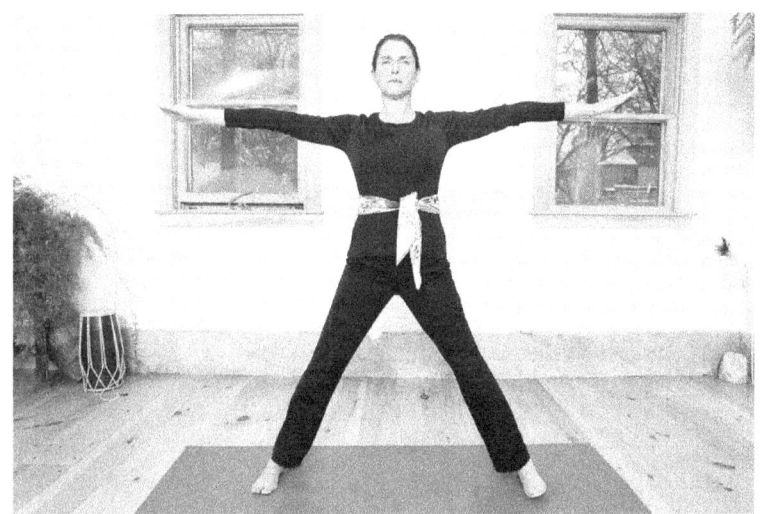

The Light of the World

John 8:12

I am the light of the world.

He that follows me shall not walk in darkness

but shall have the light of life.

How to practice

- Stand in mountain
- Take a deep breath in.
- Exhale , stepping out wide about three feet
- Be sure shoulders are over hips
- Feet face forward
- Extend arms out to the side, in line with the shoulders, parallel to the floor
- Lengthen the back of the neck.
- Radiate your light in all directions
- Receive

Variations

- Keep arms to the side
- Place arms in eagle position
- Palms in prayer pose in front of the heart
- Clasp hands behind back and do a slight backbend

Benefits

- Opens the heart
- Lengthens the entire body
- Supports arches
- Aligns spine
- Opens hips
- Reduces back pressure
- Strengthens the legs
- Increases breath capacity
- Improves circulation
- Strengthens ankles, knees, thighs

Contraindications

- Knee injuries or inflammation
- Shoulder injuries or inflammation
- Prolapsed uterus

Utthita Trikonasana

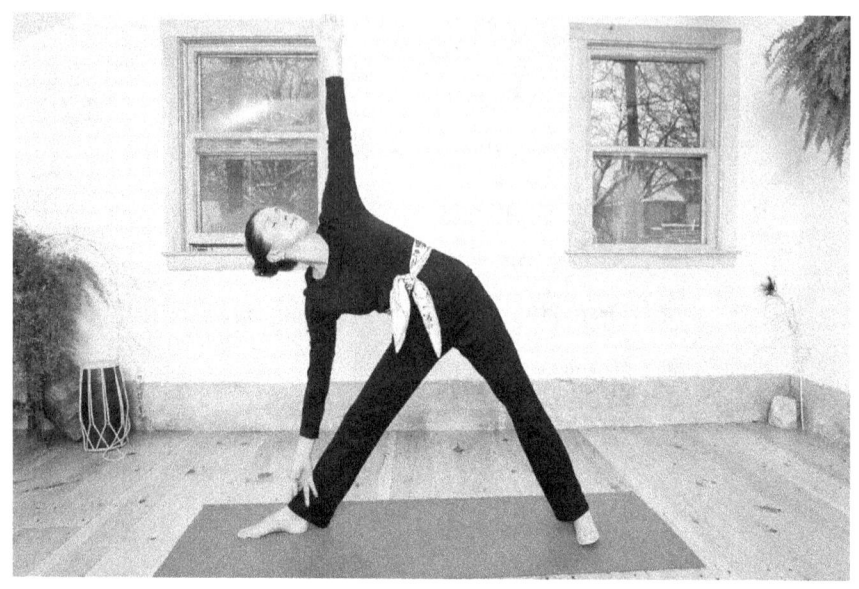

The Altogether Lovely

Song of Solomon 5:16

His mouth is most sweet, yes He is altogether lovely.

This is my Beloved; this is my friend, O daughters of Jerusalem.

How to practice

- Come to the left side of your mat in Tad asana, arms overhead.
- Step feet 3- 4' apart sideways and spread your arms into a T.
- Rotate your right hip inwards towards your pubic bone, right foot faces in about 15 degrees.
- Turn your left hip slightly out, left foot is facing straight ahead.
- Left heel lines up with the center of your right arch.
- Reach your right hip out to the right as you fold over the crease of your left hip.
- Elongate through the torso as you keep reaching
- When you have reached far enough for you, pivot your torso so the left arm reaches to the inner left leg, calf or floor
- Right arm lifts up to the sky, palms facing forward, fingers spread.
- Extend from your heart out to your fingertips
- To turn your head up , roll your chest around and then turn your head up to look at your hand
- Press into your feet to come up
- Reverse to the other side.

Variations

- Place right hand behind back
- Place right hand on right shoulder to open heart
- Extend right arm over right ear
- Switch arms when reaching to right leg.

Benefits

- Tones kidneys
- Encourages healthy digestion
- Strengthens ankles, knees
- Opens hips
- Strengthens bones
- Opens hamstrings
- Releases neck tension
- Opens heart, shoulders, upper chest area
- Helps balance

Contraindications/Cautions

- Lower back/sacrum injuries
- Groin injuries
- Weak knees
- Hyper extended knees
- Ankle breaks or sprains
- Recurrent injury in shoulders

Virabhadrasana I

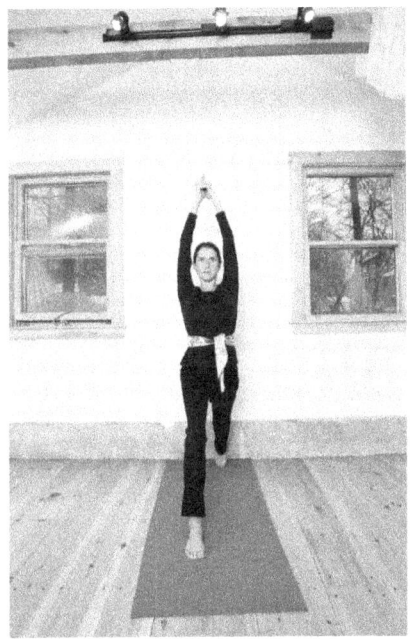

Warrior I

My Advocate

I John 2:1

My little children, these things I write to you, that you sin not.
And if any man sin, we have an advocate with the Father,
Jesus Christ the righteous.

How to practice

- Stand in Tadasana
- Step the right foot forward about 3'
- Turn the left foot in about 15 degrees
- Square hips forward
- Tuck your tailbone
- Lift ribs up off hips
- Draw navel back to the spine
- Lift arms up overhead
- Lift heart
- Step left foot to meet the right
- Step to the back of the mat
- Repeat on the other side

Variations

- Interlock hands overhead
- Arch backward
- Interlock hands behind back
- Eagle arms

Benefits

- Concentration
- Focus
- Poise
- Confidence
- Strength,
- Resilience to spine
- Bones placed properly
- Strengthens ankles, knees, thighs , hips, back, arms, shoulders, neck, Thighs, abdominals
- Prevents scoliosis
- Decongests nervous system
- Firms legs, buttocks, thighs, arms
- Stimulates digestion

Contraindications /Cautions

- High blood pressure
- Weak knees
- Inflammation in hips, shoulders, ankles, knees, abdomen
- Cardiac condition
- Neck injury

Virabhadrasana II

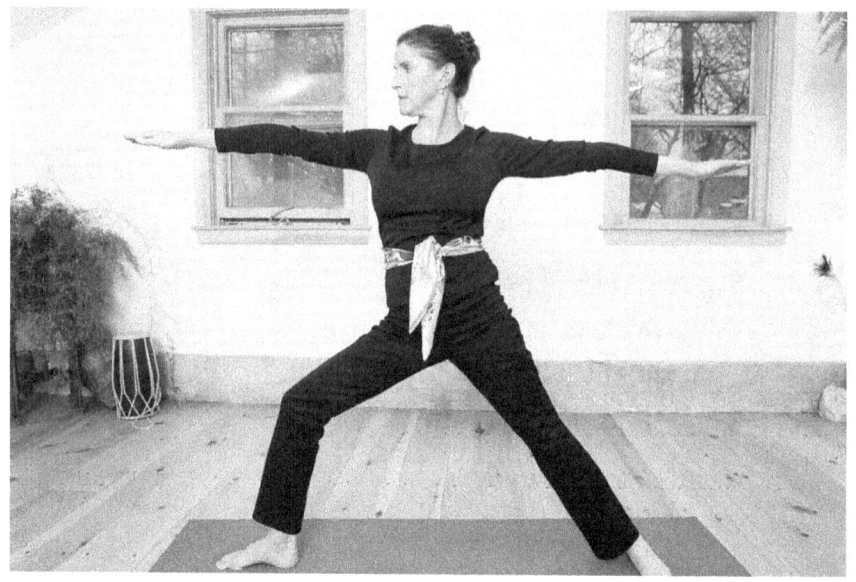

Warrior II Pose

The mediator

I Timothy 2:5

For there is one God and one mediator between God and men,

The man Jesus Christ.

How to practice

- Stand sideways in Tadasana in the center of your mat
- Step you feet wide 3 ½ feet.
- Open arms wide.
- Turn your right foot straight ahead
- Turn your left in about 15 degrees. Your left foot will follow.
- Bend your right knee to a 90 degree angle, knee parallel to the ankle.
- Line up shoulders and hips
- Arms are in line with the shoulders
- Gaze over the right fingertips
- Reverse sides

Variations

- Eagle arms
- Lift front arm to the sky, back arm to the back thigh
- Turn palms up
- Palms in prayer pose at the heart

Benefits

- Strengthens legs, ankles, knees
- Helps in treatment of prolapsed disc
- Alleviates injury to tailbone
- Relieves lower backache
- Tones kidneys
- Increases lung capacity
- Aligns spine
- Improves focus and balance
- Improves endurance

Contraindications/Cautions

- Heart disease
- Diarrhea
- Meniscus injury
- Injury to knees, ankles, lower back, or shoulders
- Neck injury
- High blood pressure

Parsvottanasana

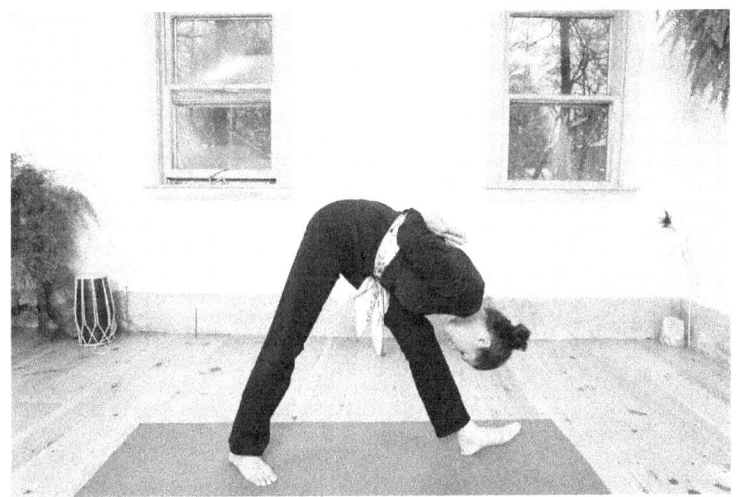

"God Hook"

A house of Defense

Psalm 31:2

Bow down thine ear to me; deliver me speedily; be thou my strong
rock, for a house of defense to save me.

How to practice

- Stand in Tadasana
- Place hands in backwards prayer hands
- Step forward with the right foot about 2 ½ feet
- Hips are facing forward
- Legs are lengthened
- Lengthen the spine
- Tuck the chin slightly
- Fold torso over the front leg
- Round lower back, tuck chin, bend front knee and release
- Switch sides

Variations

- Bend front knee
- Bend back knee
- Place hands on yoga blocks in front of the front foot

Benefits

- Corrects slooping shoulders
- Increases hip flexibility
- Relieves joint stress
- Stretches hamstrings
- Stimulates thyroid and parathyroid
- Soothes nervous system
- Relieves menstrual cramps
- Tones liver, spleen and pancreas

Contraindications/Cautions

- Pregnancy
- Shoulder injury
- Ankle injury
- Low blood pressure
- High blood pressure
- Recent abdominal surgery
- Abdominal hernia

Utkatasana

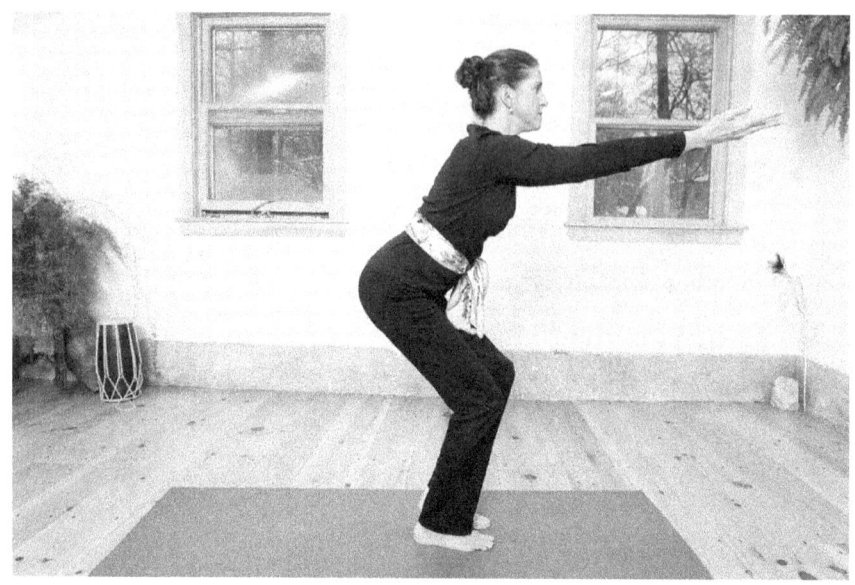

Chair Pose

A sure Foundation

Isaiah 28:16

Therefore I lay a stone in Zion
A tested stone
A precious cornerstone for a sure foundation
The one who trusts will never be dismayed.

How to practice

- Come into mountain
- Bend knees as if you were about to sit in a chair
- Keep tailbone slightly tucked
- Extend arms out in front parallel to ground or overhead, parallel to the shoulders
- Draw belly in and up
- Lift arches
- Dristi(gaze) is straight ahead

Variations

- Arms by the side
- Go on tip toes and squat all the way down, backs of thighs on backs of calves, bottom on heels
- Stand on tip toes and bend deeper
- Come into eagle arms
- Hold a strap between hands or wrap strap around forearms or upper arms
- Lean bottom against wall
- Work face to face with a partner, grabbing above wrists
- Practice sitting and getting up from a chair using abdominal muscles and quads

Benefits

- Focus, strength, power
- Blood flows more easily to hips, legs and ankles
- Can helps with arthritis in knees and ankles
- Lumbago and disc problems alleviated
- Can help increase digestion, eliminating constipation
- Abdominal toning
- More space in the diaphragm for breath
- Relieves stiffness

Contraindications/Cautions

- KNEES!!! Surgery, problems,, injuries
- shoulder surgery- have arms by side
- High blood pressure- shorter hold
- Achilles tendon injury-do only after completely healed and with great caution
- Weak ankles- very small chair pose- just a little bend in knees
- lower back injuries- Extreme caution getting OUT of pose-use wall or lean on a chair to get up

Prasarita Padottanasana

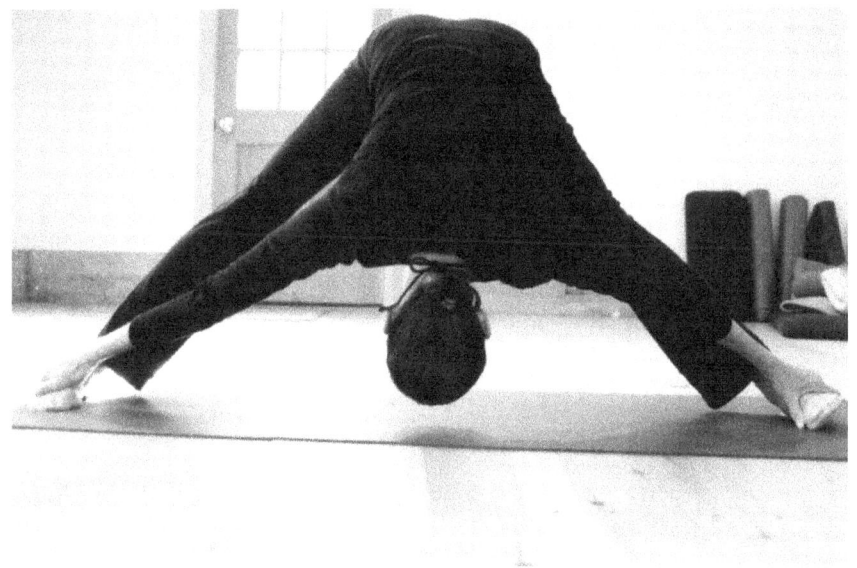

Wide-Legged Forward Bend

Root out of Dry Ground

Isaiah 53:2

For he shall grow up before me as a tender plant,

and as a root out of dry ground: he hath no from nor comeliness.

How to practice

- Stand in mountain pose
- Step or jump feet out wide 3- 3 ½ feet apart.
- Place your hands at your hips.
- Breathe in, lengthening the spine
- Press into the feet, lifting the arches
- Exhale fold at the hip creases
- Reach palms towards floor or blocks.
- Open the inner thighs as you draw feet towards each other isometrically.
- Place hands on hips as you rise up.
- Come back to mountain.

Benefits

- Benefits
- Strengthens ankles
- Stretches inner thighs
- Lengthens spine
- Clears the brain
- Tones organs
- Relaxes and opens pelvis

Contraindications

- Knee injury
- Lower back injury
- High blood pressure
- Ankle injury

Uttanasana

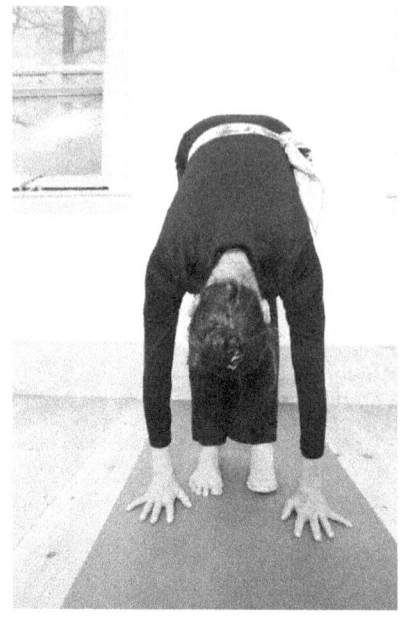

Standing Forward Bend

The Amen

Revelation 3:14

And unto the angel of the church of Laodiceans write:
These things saith the AMEN, the faithful and true witness,
the beginning of the creation of God.

How to practice

- Stand in Mountain Pose
- Place side of hands in crease of hips
- Exhale as you bend forward at hips, bending over hands
- Place hands to sides of feet
- Inhale look up, lengthening the spine, exhale drop down
- Release spine and neck down

Variations

- Grab hold of opposite elbows once you are down
- Grab big toes with index fingers and thumbs
- Take forearms behind calves and reach arms into calves, calves into arms
- Criss cross arms behind calves, then wrap hands around front of shins
- Place hastas(hands) palms up, under padas- either at fingertips or at wrists
- Place palms at wall and only go half way into forward bend- also can do with hands at edge of a chair
- Use blocks under hands

Benefits

118

- Reduces stress
- Calms mind
- Opens hamstrings
- Tones internal organs
- Improves digestion
- Energizes the spine
- Reduces anxiety

Contraindications/Cautions

- Back injury
- High Blood pressure.
- Torn hamstring
- Detached Retina

Garudhasana

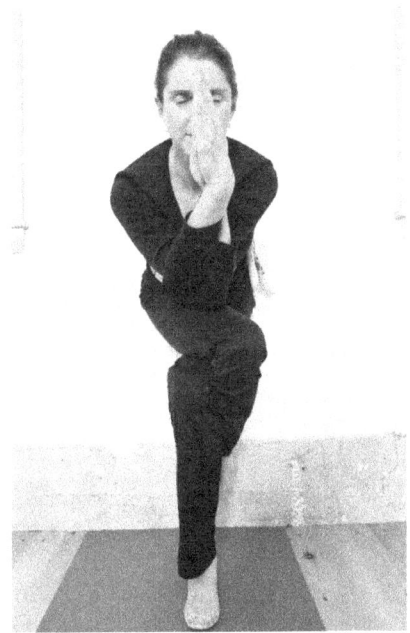

Eagle Pose

The Secret of Thy Presence

Psalm 31:20

Thou shalt hide them in the secret of the presence from the pride of
man: thou shalt keep them secretly in a pavilion from the strife of
tongues.

How to practice

- Stand in Mountain
- Invite the left leg over the right thigh and wrap the left foot around the back
- Open the arms wide as you inhale, squawk like an eagle. Exhale. Cross the left elbow under the right elbow
- Sink down as if about to sit in a chair
- Press in to the standing leg. Slightly straighten, release the arms and stand upright.
- Go to the other side

Variations

- Place hands in prayer pose
- Fold hands over elbows
- Lean against a wall

Benefits

- Improves focus and concentration
- Stretches calves
- Creates balance in the body
- Reduces shoulder tension

Contraindications/Cautions

- Knee injuries
- Shoulder injuries

Parabola

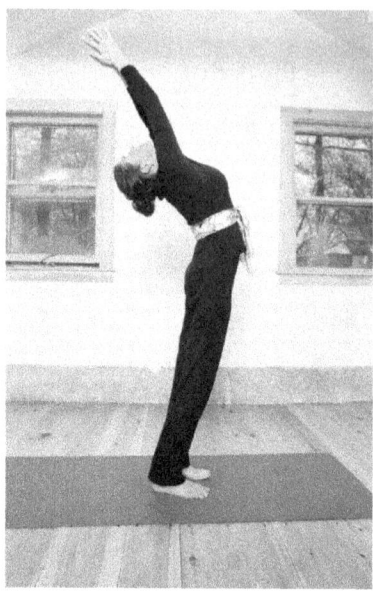

Morning Star

2 Peter 1:19

And we have the word of the prophets made more certain and you will
do well to pay attention to it, as to a light shining in a dark place until
the day dawns and the morning star rises in your hearts.

How to practice

- Stand in Mountain
- Interlock Hands and raise them above your head
- Be sure to draw tailbone and pubic bone towards each other first, lift belly under navel, then arch back

Variations

- As you interlock hands, bend at elbows to cradle head and arch whole body back
- Normally you inhale as you extend and exhale as you drop back, but this may cause undue stress on lower back and knees, so try to reverse the pattern to allow greater support of the body in backbend
- Place a block between the thighs
- Stand back to wall about 2' and reach hands back, finger tips pointing down

Benefits

- Creates huge breath capacity
- Stretches entire body, energizing it
- Develops greater body awareness of personal edge
- Elongates the spine, creating space between each vertebrae
- Tones kidneys
- Develops balance and strength
- Stronger core
- Prepares body for other backbends
- Detoxifies nervous system

Contraindications

- Weak knees
- Shoulder injuries
- Vertigo
- Lower back problems- proceed with Great caution

Adho Mukha Svanasana

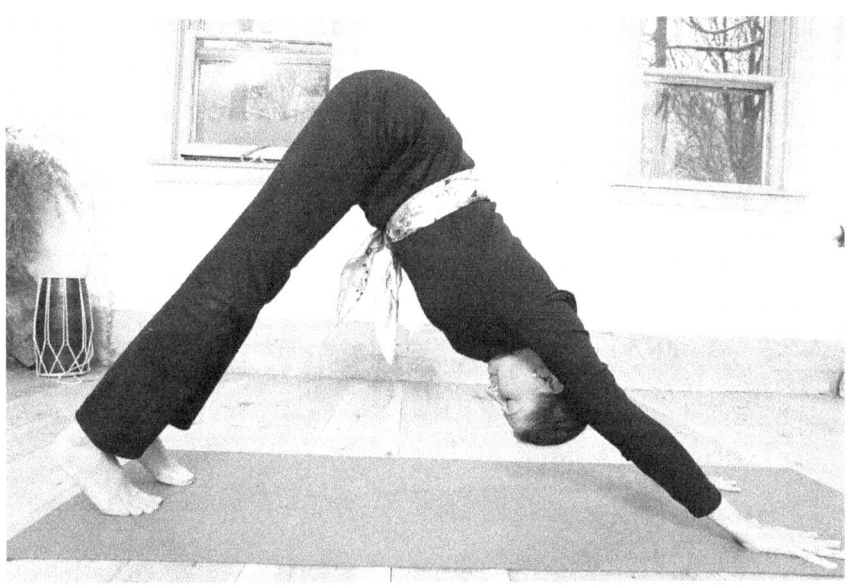

Downward-Facing Dog

Servant

Isaiah 42:1

Behold my Servant, whom I uphold: mine elect, in whom my soul
delighteth; I have put my Spirit upon Him.

How to practice

- Start in table position, with hands firmly placed under shoulders, and knees under hips.

- Press into palms and fingers, the mound of the thumb and index finger especially

- Roll the armpits forward and the head of the arm bones back.

- Make the belly flush to the spine

- Curl the toes under, breathe in , exhale and press into a downward V with hips raised

- Keep hips lifted with bent knees.

- Create a loop from the top of the tailbone down the back of the legs through the back heels, under the body to the heels of the hands and fingertips.

- Continue to press firmly into hands as you lengthen the spine and the legs.

- Dristi is slightly in towards heart

- Release by bending the knees back into table

Variations

- Practice with fisted hands
- Practice with palms pressing into a wall
- Practice on forearms

Benefits

- Lengthening of the spine
- Calm and decongest nervous system
- Greater flow to lymphatic system
- Stimulates circulation
- Stimulates and regulates the glands, in particular the thyroid, hyperthyroid, pineal, pituitary
- Tones face
- Stimulates hair growth
- Can help with sciatica
- Helps stimulate brain function

Contraindications/Cautions

- Problem knees, hamstrings, severe sciatica
- Unmedicated High blood pressure
- Detached retina
- Conjunctivitis
- Injury or surgery in shoulders

Bhujangasana

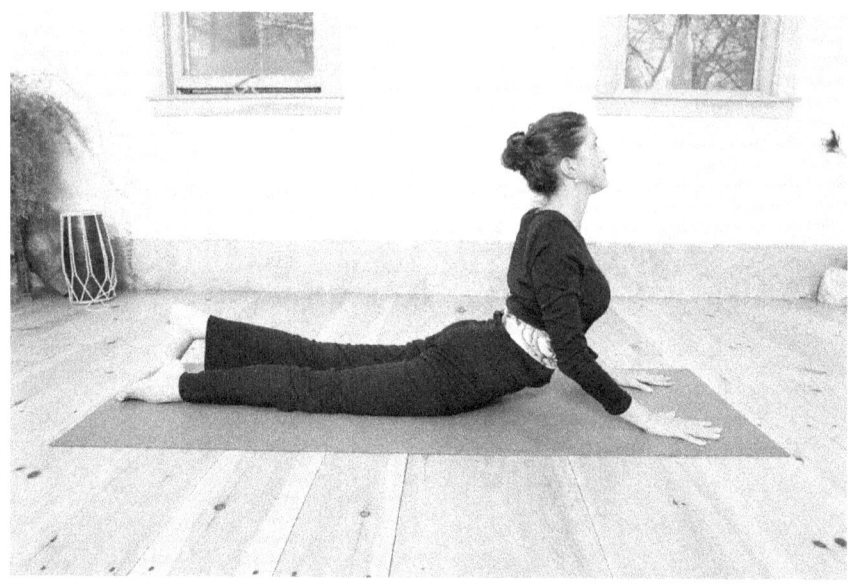

Cobra Pose

Serpent in the Wilderness

John 3:14

And as Moses lifted up the serpent in the wilderness, even so must the Son of man be lifted up.

How to practice

- Lie on belly, legs extended behind you, tailbone slightly tucked under, pubic bone triangle firmly anchored in the floor. Lift the navel in and up under the ribs slightly

- Bend elbows and place hands parallel to nipple area. Hug elbows close to the body

- Inhale press out through the toes and press tops of feet on the floor.

- Press into pubic bone and tops of legs.

- Inhale press into palms to lengthen arms and lift chest off the floor. Puff chest forward as you lengthen and strengthen the back muscles.

- Lift throat out of collarbone and gaze forward.

- Release and turn cheek to one side.

Variations

Place forearms on the ground

Benefits

- Kidney toner
- Strengthens wrists, arms, shoulders, muscles in the back
- Nourishes the spine and tones nervous system
- Opens chest for easier breathing
- Contracts dorsal muscles in lumbar spine.
- Strengthens abdominals
- Helps relieve cramps with menses
- Extremely beneficial to tonify uterus and ovaries.
- Lengthens side body

Contraindications/Cautions

- Pregnancy after three months- don't do.
- Lower back injury
- Abdominal surgery
- Ongoing inflammation in shoulders- do baby cobra instead.
- Weak back muscles- practice baby cobra or abdominal curls

Salabhasana

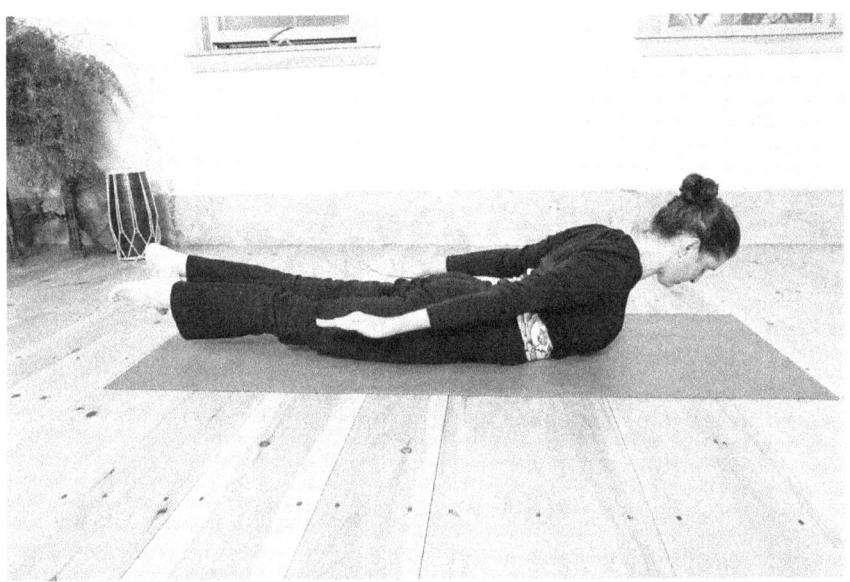

Locust Pose

God in the Midst

Psalm 46:5

God is in the midst of her: she shall not be moved.

God shall help her and that right early.

How to practice

- Lie on the belly with feet close and arms, palms down, along the side of the torso.
- Chin rests on the floor.
- Drop the coccyx slightly to the pubic bone with a small tuck.
- Inhale and lengthen from the navel to the crown and the navel to the toes.
- Draw the thigh bones and shin bones up to the back of the legs.
- Press into the palms and pubic bone and extend through your toes, lifting the legs off the floor just a few inches.
- This pose is about length, rather than height. Imagine trying to reach the back wall with your toes.
- Release the legs to the floor, relax and receive the pose.'

Variations

- Only do the lower body
- Only do the upper torso
- Interlock hands behind sacrum and pull back and up as you rise

Benefits

- Lumbar spine strengthener
- Abdominal strengthener
- Blood flow to the sacral region
- Flushed toxins from the kidneys
- Strengthens abdominal muscles
- By releasing venous pressure in the legs, can reduce varicose veins
- Tones endocrine, nervous and digestive system
- Buttock muscles strengthened.
- Elongates body to improve posture
- Energizes the back body

Contraindications/Cautions

- With weak back muscles do 3-4 repetitions to strengthen.
- With head and neck problems, place rolled blanket under the head
- Not to be done if more than 3 months pregnant.
- No for recent abdominal surgery
- No for recent or chronic inflammation or serious injury to lower back, spine, legs, arms or shoulders.

Garbhasana

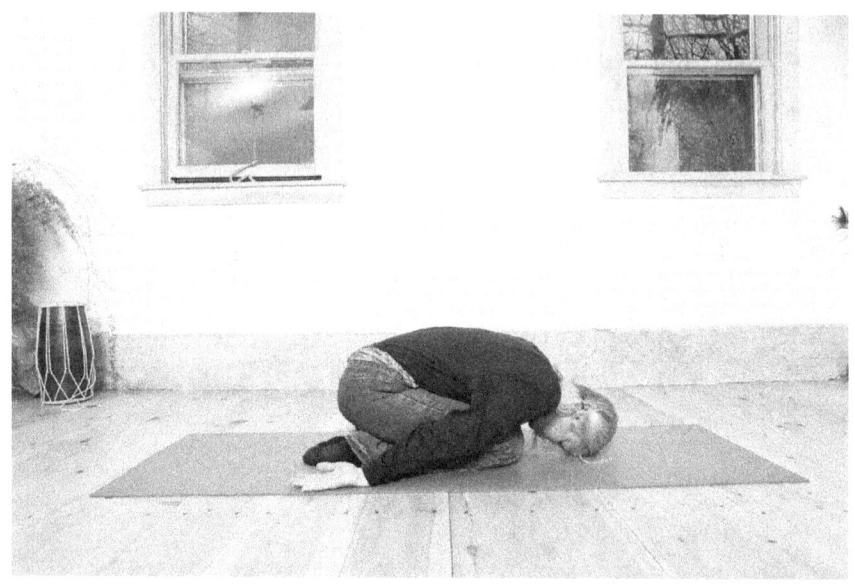

Child's Pose

The First Begotten

Colossians 1:15-17

He is the image of the invisible God, the firstborn over all creation. For by him all things were created: things in heaven and on earth, visible and invisible, whether thrones or powers or rulers or authorities: all things were created by him and for him. He is before all things and in him all things hold together.

How to practice

- Come to all fours with hands directly beneath shoulders
- Take a breath in, Sit back on heels
- Bend at hips and fold torso over thighs, chest to knees
- Rest forehead to ground
- Hands towards feet, palms up. Breathe.
- To release, slide hands under shoulders and press up into sitting position, Rock hips to one side and stretch legs out in front

Variations

- Extend arms in front
- Extend arms in front and turn palms face up

Benefits

- Counter stretch for backbends.
- Soothes pelvic bowl.
- Calms the mind

Contraindications/Cautions

- Knee sensitivity
- Stiff hips and legs
- Head trauma or high blood pressure

Dandasana

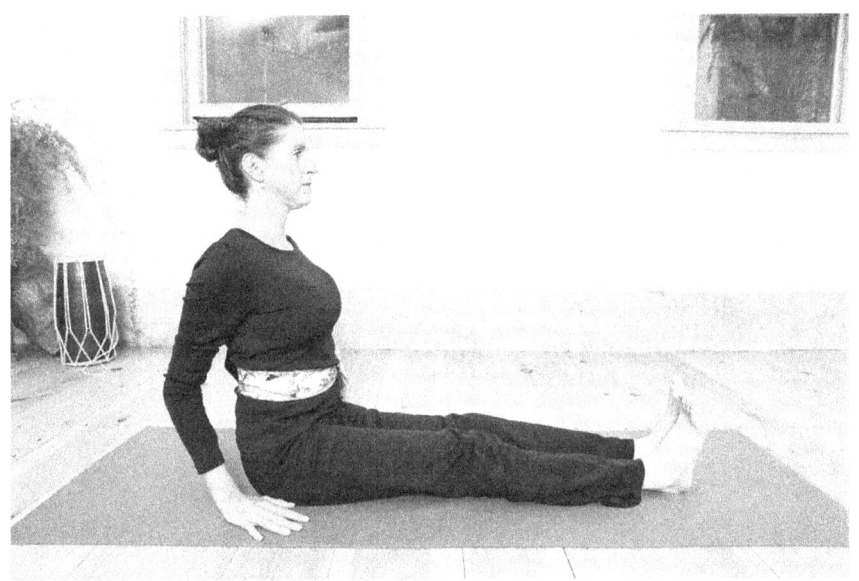

Staff Pose

Rod

Isaiah 11:1

And there shall come forth a rod out of the stem of Jesse and a Branch shall grow out of his roots.

How to practice

- Sit on the floor with your legs outstretched.
- Be sure your spine is upright and the neck is directly over the spine.
- Hands are to your side, palms down.
- Flex the feet. Breathe.

Variations

- Hands in prayer pose
- Sit on the edge of a pillow to roll hips forward for tight hamstrings

Benefits

- Hamstring opener
- Opens back side of the body
- clears brain
- relaxes heart
- stimulates peristalsis

Contraindications

- acute sciatica
- back injury or inflammation

Maha Mudra

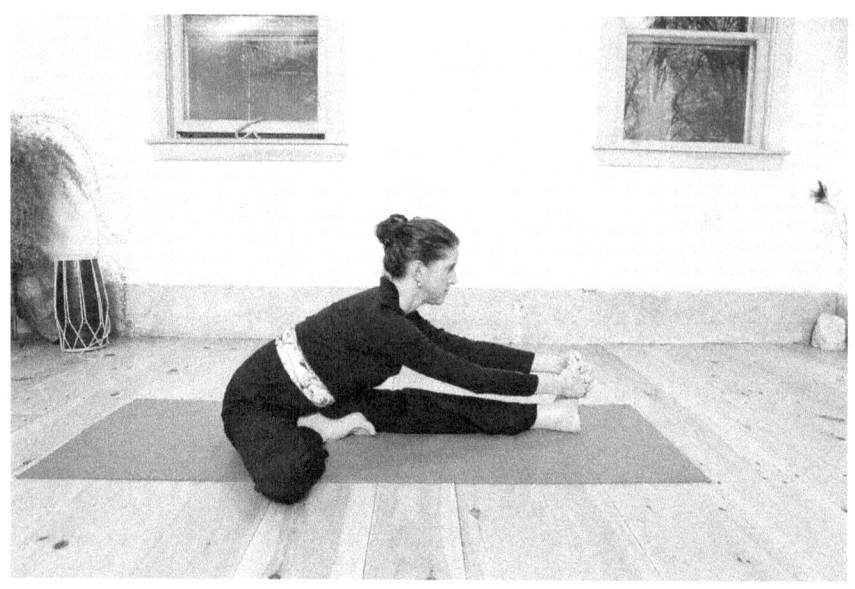

The Great Seal

My Hiding Place

Psalm 32:7

Thou art my hiding place: thou shalt preserve me from trouble; Thou shalt compass me about with songs of deliverance. Selah.

How to practice

- Sit in Staff Pose
- Flex feet
- Bend right knee, placing right foot inside left thigh or calf
- Lengthen spine as you extend forward
- Keep heart lifted
- Grab hold of right foot
- Reverse sides

Variations

- Hold strap around foot of extended leg
- Place bent knee on a pillow
- Sit on the edge of a pillow , rolling hips forward , for hip balance

Benefits

- Balances chakras
- Stretches the back body
- Opens hamstrings
- Improves digestion
- Increases energy
- Invigorates the mind

Contraindications

- Lower back injury
- Sciatica
- Hamstring injury
- Torn Achilles

l

Ardha Matsyendrasana

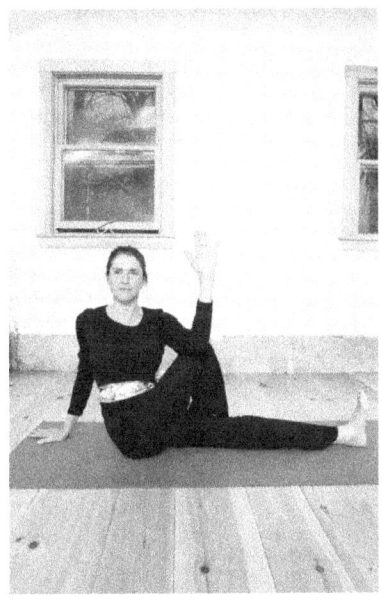

Half Lord of the Fishes Pose

Covenant

Isaiah 42:6

I the Lord have called thee in to righteousness, and will hold thine hand, and will keep thee, and give thee for a covenant of the people, for a light to the Gentiles.

How to practice

- Sit with legs outstretched. Draw left knee into chest and cross left foot over right thigh to right
- Inhale, Lengthen spine, Hug left knee with right arm, Stretch left arm out
- Reach left arm around to left buttock, Inhale. Stretch tall. Exhale. Twist.
- Release and do other side

Variations

- Place elbow to the inside of the bent knee
- Twist in the opposite direction if you are pregnant
- Bend extended leg , placing foot under opposite buttocks

Benefits

- Tones inner organs
- Flushes the spine
- Relieves menstrual cramps reduces stiffness in the joints
- Creates vitality in the body
- Stimulates digestion

Contraindications/Cautions

- Spinal injury
- Back injury
- Herniated discs
- Lower back problems
- Recent abdominal surgery

Paschimottanasana

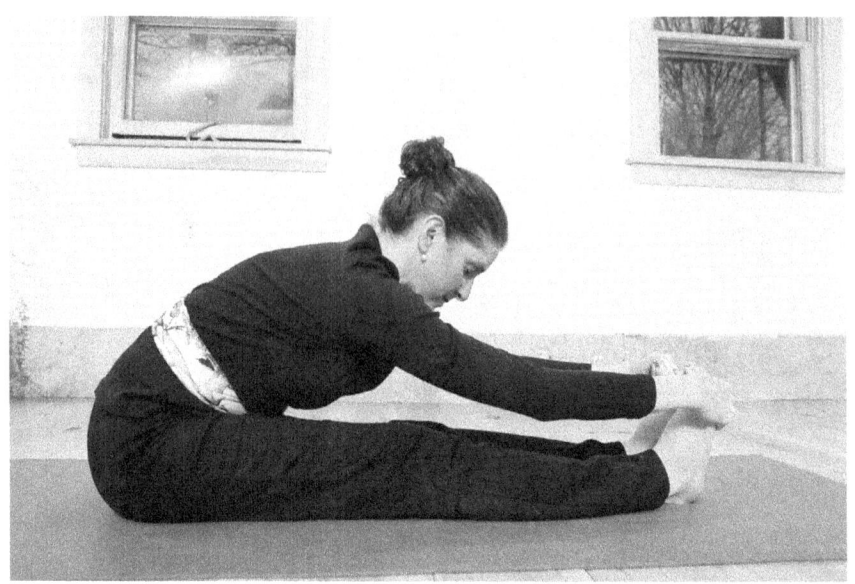

Seated Forward Bend

Shepherd

Psalm 23:1

The Lord is my shepherd; I shall not want.

How to practice

- Sit in Staff Pose
- Inhale, Lift arms to the sky
- Exhale. Roll at hips. Reach arms forward towards toes.
- Bend forward
- Release by pressing in to legs
- Reach arms along side of body
- Sit up tall

Variations

- Place hands on yoga blocks on either side of hips
- Grab hold of a yoga strap around the feet

Benefits

- Hamstring opener
- Opens back side of the body,
- clears brain
- relaxes heart
- stimulates peristalsis

Contraindications/Cautions

- acute sciatica
- back injury or inflammation

149

Upavistha Konasana

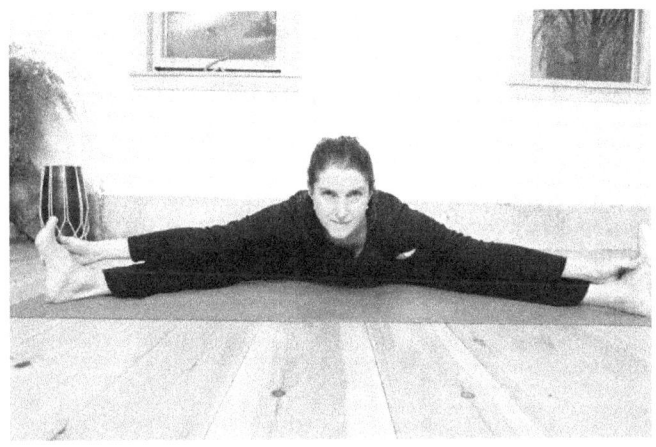

Wide-Angle Seated Forward Bend

Holy One

Psalm 99:5

Exalt the Lord our God and worship at his footstool. He is holy.

How to practice

- Sit with legs outstretched in a "V"
- Inhale, Grab hold of big toes
- Exhale. Roll at hips forward with the torso
- Inhale, Lengthen spine.
- Exhale, Fold forward.
- Inhale. Press into legs. Lift back up.
- Release

Variations

- Place hands on yoga blocks in front
- Lean on forearms
- Bend knees slightly
- Grab hold of each foot with a yoga strap

Benefits

- Stimulates circulation in pelvis
- Opens and stretches hamstrings

Contraindications

- lower back injury
- sciatica

Setu Bandha Sarvangasana

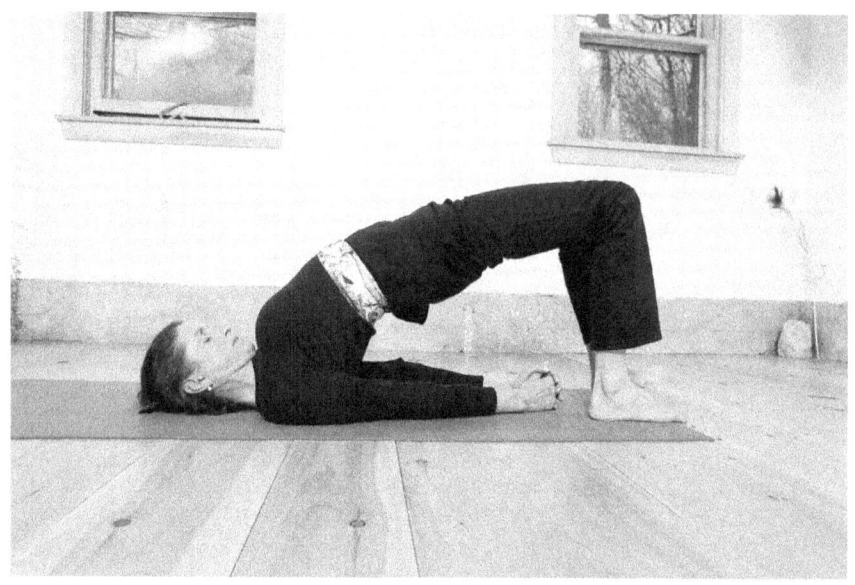

Bridge Pose

Living Bread

John 6:50-51

I am the living bread that came down from heaven. If anyone eats of this bread, he will live forever. This bread is my flesh, which I will give for the life of the world.

How to practice

- Reach hands down towards toes, palms down
- Tuck chin towards chest slightly
- Plant feet firmly beneath knees, toes facing forward
- Inhale. Tuck tailbone under
- Exhale. Lift belly up to sky
- Roll shoulder blades under back
- Interlock fingers and squeeze palms together
- Inhale. Exhale. Release

Variations

- Place a yoga block under the lower back
- Wrap a yoga strap around the lower calves and reach for the strap with both hands

Benefits

- Opens chest and heart
- Strengthens ankles
- Opens hips

Contraindications/Cautions

- Lower back or neck injury
- High blood pressure

Salamba Sarvangasana

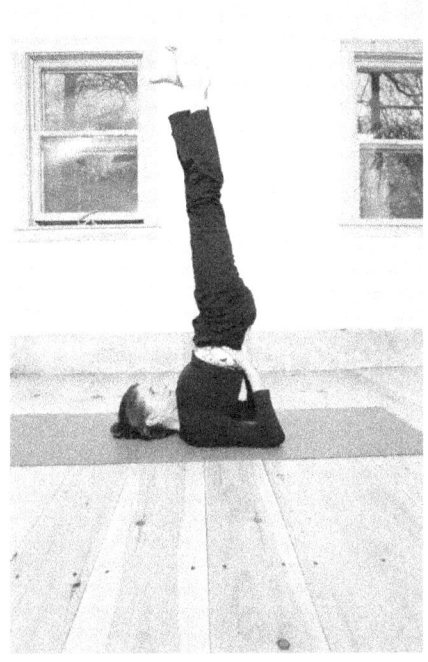

Supported Shoulderstand

The End of the Law

Romans 10:4

Christ is the end of the Law so that there may be righteousness for everyone who believes.

How to practice

- Lie on back, hands to sides
- Bend knees in to chest
- Support buttocks and lower back with hands
- Stretch legs up to the sky. Flicker like a candle
- Bend knees to chest and release

Variations

- Tilt hips and form a V with legs into a half shoulderstand
- Place a yoga block underneath the lower back
- Lean back body against a wall
- Keep bottom on the floor and lean legs against the wall

157

Benefits

- Helps with hair growth
- Calms brain
- Relaxes heart
- Relieves headaches
- Reduces varicose veins
- A natural facial
- Relaxes the colon

Contraindications/Cautions

- neck and shoulder injury,
- high blood pressure,
- extreme low blood pressure
- eye conditions such as detached retina
- glaucoma, eye infection
- menses
- severe thyroid conditions
- menstruation

Matsyasana

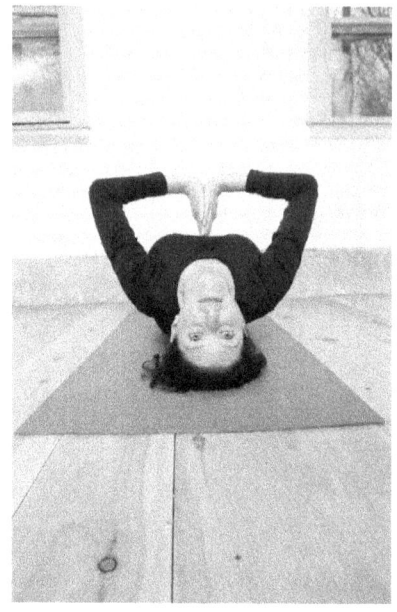

Fish Pose

Fountain of Living Water

John 4:14

Whoever drinks the water I give him will never thirst. Indeed the water I give him will become in him a spring of water welling up to eternal life.

How to practice

- Lie on back. Legs outstretched. Slide hand under buttocks or legs, palms down
- Bend elbows, Press in to forearms, Lift head off floor. Arch back.
- Gently place crown of head on the floor
- Slide head down
- Walk arms out from underneath

Variations

- Place yoga block lengthwise under mid back
- Lie mid back over a pillow or bolster with another pillow under back of head

Benefits

- Spinal flexibility
- Chest opener
- Stimulates thyroid
- Can help prevent diabetes by stimulating pancreas
- Grief release

Contraindications

- Weak neck and back
- Neck and shoulder injury
- Insomnia

Journal Questions

What does sitting in the consciousness of God mean to you?

What yoga pose resonates most with you? Why?

What yoga pose is most challenging for you? Why?

See each of these two poses as Bible verses. What is the message of each of these poses for you?

What does it mean to embody Christ on the planet?

Relaxation

&

Creative

Visualization

Relaxation Pose, or Sivasana, is the most wonderful gift that comes at the end of Yoga Practice. It can be incredibly rewarding and deeply satisfying. As you rest on your back you receive the blessings of your practice, the fruit of your labor. Many times relaxation pose can offer you opportunities to hear your body's messages more clearly. Relaxation has been studied for many years, and they can now document decreased blood pressure, increase in immune system, released tension in muscles, nerves strengthened. Relaxation has even been known to reduce glucose levels in diabetic patients.

Relaxation techniques are simple. Be sure you feel comfortable, not distracted by bright lights, loud music, cold air, or super hard surfaces.

Sivasana

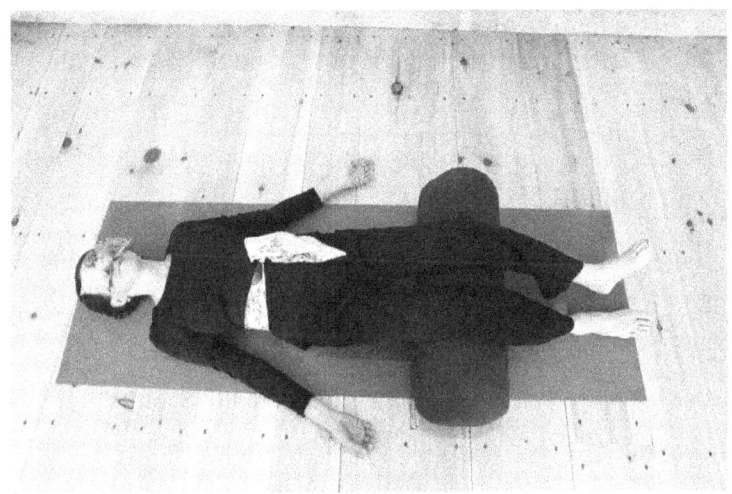

Relaxation Pose

I surrender

1 Corinthians 15:31

Brothers, by the right to be proud which the Messiah Yeshua our Lord gives me, I solemnly tell you that I die every day.

How to practice

- Stand in easy mountain
- Take a deep breath in, breathe out as you roll down to the ground
- Bend your knees and sit, then stretch your legs out as you lie on your back.
- Bend your elbows, and then push the upper arms into the ground as you draw the shoulder blades towards each other more to open the chest.
- Place Hands by your hips, palms open and relaxed.
- Let your feet fall out to the side
- Close your eyes
- Relax your jaw
- Relax your body completely, bringing all your attention softly to your breath at first
- Eventually let even that focus go.
- Let your thoughts float away like little clouds
- Surrender to the pose.

Variations

- Place a bolster or pillow underneath your knees
- Lie on your belly
- Place one hand on the belly, one hand on the heart
- Elevate the head if you have high blood pressure or other heart issues

Benefits

- Stress reduction
- Balances all body systems
- Gives body a chance to receive good prana
- Nervous system recalibrated
- Soothes the mind

Contraindications

- PTSD may cause re-triggering
- Congestive heart failure

Relaxation Techniques

Contraction and release

This can be done with the whole body contracting at once on the inhale and then letting go on the exhale, or contracting and releasing each individual body parts (usually starting with the feet) and telling each body part to contract on the inhale and relax and let go on the exhale.

Heavy body

Allow the body to feel heavy, sometimes even using a prop of a weight on the belly. As you relax more and more in to the posture, the body becomes lighter and lighter. Feel burdens lifted.

Creative Visualization. This can address sickness, stress, and a difficult task. As you breathe in and out imagine tension releasing, visualize first the "problem", embracing it fully and bringing your compassionate breath to it, then visualize the "problem" dissolving. Surround it with the love of Christ. Send a color to it, like White Light.

Affirmation. As you go deeper in to relaxation and letting go, the deep reservoir of peace that comes in to the space is palpable. This is Sacred Unity. Silently repeat an affirmation to yourself three times before complete surrender. A wonderful affirmation is the following-"I *am whole and fully present*". Or "I *live in constant grace.*"

Yoga Nidra- Lie on the back. Gently tell each part of the body to relax. Breathe deeply. Be conscious of your body as you feel each body part relaxing. Allow those body parts to relax even more as you deeply breathe in to these places. Let the thoughts of the mind have roundness to them- let them lose their sharpness, to the point where they drift away like clouds.

"Come *to me, all you who are weary and burdened and I will give you rest. Take my yoke upon you and learn from me, for I am gentle and humble in heart, and you will find REST for your souls."* Matthew 11:28-29.

Being the earth. As you lie on your back, allow your body to begin to melt in to the floor. Feel as if there is no longer any line of separation between you and the earth. Become the earth. Feel your body as a part of the entire earth, because you are.

Let go completely.

Thy will be done, Lord. Thy will be done.

How to come out of Savasana

- Take deep breaths
- Place one hand on heart and one hand on belly
- Focus on your breath
- Open your ears. Become more aware of sounds in the room
- Rub your palms together , then cup your eyes
- Open your eyes as you pull hands away
- Circle wrists and ankles
- Move knees and hips
- Roll head side to side as you follow your breath
- Hug knees into chest as you rock side to side
- Stretch entire body
- Roll to your right side- Why? To relax the heart muscle and help stimulate the colon
- Press into your left hand and roll up to sit.

Relaxation can last anywhere from 5-30 minutes. You can end your practice with Nadi Shodhana or silent meditation. Enjoy the benefits of this restorative practice.

Meditation

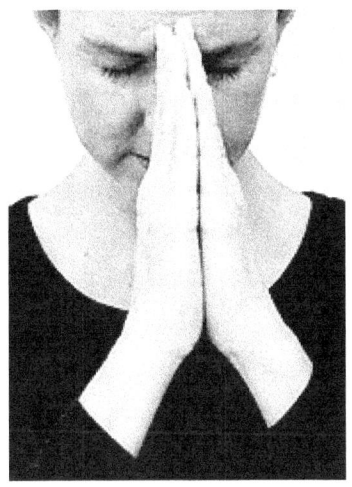

Meditation is turning inward to see God. It is the practice of Dhyana, one of the eight limbs of Raja Yoga. Meditation has many of the same benefits as relaxation pose: increased mental clarity, reduced blood pressure, stress reduction, peace. As you sit in meditation, withdrawing your senses from the outside world, you discover an inside world that can be just as noisy. The practice of meditation stills the inner and outer noise.

The gift of meditation is the ability to be present, to be totally in the magnificent now, with no agenda! The sense of timelessness can take over as you delve further and further in to the depths of God.

In order to meditate at optimum, be sure your space is uncluttered, warm enough, comfortable, and free of noise and bright lights. Of course if that is not possible, simply shutting the eyes can begin to tune out the outer world. Sit cross legged, on a chair or in lotus position, with the spine erect and the knees below the hips. If the knees are above the hips, sit on a pillow or a few pillows. If you are tired, sit against a wall. It is best to be sitting, though, so the energy can flow freely up and down the central nadi (river) of the body, the spine.

Ways of meditating

- Meditate on a word or phrase, such as Peace, or Jesus.

- Repeat a mantra such as Allah-Ha or Hallelujah.

- Focus on the in and out breath to get grounded.

- Bring your attention to the heart, open it and connect with God and with others.

- Meditate on the brow point for wisdom and clarity.

- Sit and BE the Witness.

- Meditate on the breath going in and going out, rising in and falling down, with a mantra- "Breathing in I am breathing in, Breathing out I am breathing out."

- Meditate on a single mantra with mala beads or a rosary.

- Meditate on God's word, reading it aloud or silently to yourself, and then allowing the Word to infuse your whole being.

- Sit in a comfortable position while listening to sacred music and allowing that music to fill your cells with vibrant sound.

Jesus went off in to the wilderness for 40 days of prayer, fasting and meditation.

Some great verses to meditate on are found in Psalms:

"Blessed is the (wo) man whose delight is in the law of the Lord, and his Law (s) he meditates day and night. (S)He is like a tree planted by streams of water, which yields its fruit in season and whose leaf does not wither. Whatever (s) he does prospers" **Psalm 1:1-3.**

"The commands of the Lord are radiant, giving light to the eyes. The ordinances of the Lord are sure and altogether righteous, more precious than gold, sweeter than honey." **Psalm 19:9-10.**

A Meditation Practice

The following is an exercise in meditation. You will need to record yourself first. Then find a comfortable sitting position. Allow yourself a few minutes of sitting silently to grow accustomed to your space and your experience. In the background hear the names of God being repeated over and over.

Here is a list of the mantras to be repeated for up to 30 minutes:

God, Christ, Holy Spirit, Yahweh, Jehovah, Adonai, Shekinah, El Shaddai, EL Eliyon, Elohim, I am , Love, Jesus, Eoshoa, Y;shua, Soul, Divine Mother, Mighty I am , Presence, Rock, Wonderful, Counselor, Messiah, Emmanuel, Alpha and Omega, Everlasting Light, King of Kings , Lion of Judah, Lamb, Great Shepherd, Friend, Door, Gate, Dwelling Place, King of Peace, Foundation, Holy, Bread of life, Bridegroom, Lord, Bright Morning Star, Firstborn, Bread of Life, Living God, Light, the Word, My Hiding Place.

Allow these sacred words to penetrate your being. Sit in silence. Receive in the soles of your feet, the palms of your hands, the mind, the body, the heart. Receive God in every fiber of your being. Selah.

Songs

&

Prayers

The following is a list of songs, prayers, mantras and chants which can be used in Christ-centered Yoga.

Doxology

Praise God from whom all Blessings Flow
Praise Him all creatures here below
Praise Him above the heavenly hosts
Praise Father, Son and Holy Ghost

Pace

Dona Nobis Pacem.
Give us Peace

Be Thou My Vision

Be Thou my Vision, O Lord of my heart;
Naught be all else to me, save that Thou art
Thou my best Thought, by day or by night,
Waking or sleeping, Thy presence my light.

Be Thou my Wisdom, and Thou my true Word;
I ever with Thee and Thou with me, Lord;
Thou my great Father, I Thy true son;
Thou in me dwelling, and I with Thee one.

Be Thou my battle Shield, Sword for the fight;
Be Thou my Dignity, Thou my Delight;
Thou my soul's Shelter, Thou my high Tower:
Raise Thou me heavenward, O Power of my power.

Riches I heed not, nor man's empty praise,
Thou mine Inheritance, now and always:
Thou and Thou only, first in my heart,
High King of heaven, my Treasure Thou art.

High King of heaven, my victory won,
May I reach heaven's joys, O bright heaven's Sun!
Heart of my own heart, whatever befalls,
still be my Vision, O Ruler of all.

Dallán Forgaill, Irish Traditional

Crown Him with Many Crowns

Crown Him with Many Crowns
The Lamb upon His throne
Hark how the heavenly anthem drowns
All music but its own
Awake my soul and sing
Of Him who died for thee
And hail Him as the Matchless King
Through all Eternity

Matthew Bridges, 1852, Godfrey Thring, 1874. George Elvey, 1868

All hail the power of Jesus name

All hail the power of Jesus name
Let angels prostrate fall
Bring forth the royal diadem
And crown Him Lord of all
Bring forth the royal diadem
And crown Him Lord of all
Edward Perronet

Prayers

All shall be well and all shall be well and all manner of thing shall be well. ***Julian of Norwich***

Therefore, this is how you shall pray;
Our heavenly Father, hallowed is thy name
Your kingdom is come. Your will is done.
As in heaven so also on earth.
Give us bread for the our daily need.
And leave us serene
Just as we also allowed others serenity
And do not pass us through trial
Except separate us from the evil one.
For Yours is the Kingdom, the Power and the Glory
To the end of the universe, of all universes.
      Amen. *Y'shua*

Victor Alexander, Aramaic New Testament, 1998

Saint Patrick's Breastplate

I bind myself today
The Strong name of the Trinity
By invocation of the same
The Three in One and the One in Three
I bind this to me to me forever
By power of faith, Christ's incarnation
His baptism in Jordan River
His death on cross for my salvation
His bursting from the spiced tomb
His riding up the heavenly way
His coming at the day of doom
I bind unto myself today
I bind unto myself today
The virtues of the star-lit heaven
The glorious suns life –giving ray
The whiteness of the moon at even
The flashing of the lightning free
The whirling wind's tempestuous shocks
The stable earth, the deep salt sea
Around the old eternal rocks

Christ be with me, Christ within me
Christ behind me, Christ before me
Christ beside me, Christ to win me
Christ to comfort and restore me
Christ beneath me, Christ above me
Christ in Quiet, Christ in Danger
Christ in hearts of all that love me

Christ in mouth of friend and stranger

I bind unto myself the Name
The Strong Name of the Trinity
By invocation of the same
The Three in One and One in Three
Of whom all nature hath creation
Eternal Father, Spirit, Word
Praise to the Lord of My salvation
Salvation is of Christ the Lord.

Traditional

Alternate prayer of Saint Patrick

I arise today
Through the strength of heaven,
Light of sun
Radiance of moon
Splendor of fire
Speed of lightning
Swiftness of Wind
Depth of sea
Stability of earth
Firmness of Rock

Traditional

Ancient Yoga Prayer

May the Divine Protect us while we are together
May all obstacles be removed which stand in the way
Of our understanding the truth that all is One:
And that there is no division or separation between us
May we grasp this understanding with full comprehension
And without doubt so that all misunderstanding
Is dissolved within us
May we not cherish hatred, anger or displeasure
May our hearts be full of love
May perfect friendship reign between us
May the space around us be from fear
May the East and the West, North and South, be free of fear
May the earth be free of fear
May be all unite in one fearless friendship.

Traditional

Prayer of Jabez

Oh that you would bless me
And enlarge my territory
Let your hand be with me
And keep me from harm
So that I will be free from pain
And God granted his request

NIV, I Chronicles 4:10

Bio

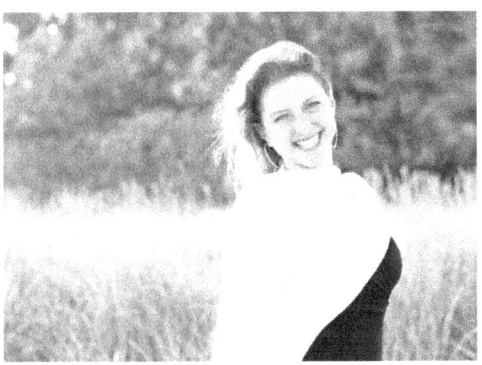

Marsha Therese Danzig, M.ED Harvard, RYT 500, is a pioneer in the fields of yoga and wellness. She is the founder of Color Me Yoga for Children, Yoga for Amputees, and Pediatric Yoga. She is the author of Fierce Joy, a memoir about choosing joy in the face of suffering, as well as numerous other children's books and yoga products. She is a storyteller, healer and spiritual teacher whose mission is to help people remember their freedom and heal their sense of separation. Her websites are www.colormeyoga.com , www.fiercejoy.net, www.yogaforamputees.com

Contact:

To book Marsha for conferences, trainings, keynote speeches and workshops, contact
marsha@fiercejoy.net

Order the complete audio set:

www.cdbaby.com/cd/marshatheresedanzig

I have loved you with an everlasting love.....